THE PHILOSOPHY OF SHAOLIN KEMPO KARATE

A Journey Towards Mastery: From Basic Principles to Advanced Techniques

KAMERON JALEN

Table of Contents

Introduction

A hybrid martial art, Shaolin Kempo Karate is a combination of techniques and principles from a variety of different martial arts, including traditional Chinese Shaolin Kung Fu, Japanese Karate, and other styles of martial arts. The purpose of this method is to provide a holistic approach to self-defense, physical fitness, and personal development strategies.

Shaolin Kempo Karate was developed in the late 20th century. Villari, a martial artist with experience in multiple disciplines, sought to create a system that blended the best aspects of different martial arts. The name "Shaolin Kempo Karate" reflects its diverse influences:

• **Shaolin:** Refers to the ancient Shaolin Temple in China, renowned for its martial arts tradition.

- **Kempo (Kenpo):** A Japanese term meaning "law of the fist," often used to describe Chinese martial arts techniques adapted in Japan.

- **Karate:** A Japanese martial art emphasizing striking techniques like punches, kicks, and knee strikes.

Key Components:

- **Striking:** Shaolin Kempo Karate incorporates powerful strikes from Karate, including punches, kicks, elbows, and knees. These techniques are designed for both offense and defense.

- **Blocking:** The system includes various blocking techniques to deflect or absorb attacks, protecting the practitioner from harm.

• **Grappling and Joint Locks:** Borrowing from Chinese martial arts and Jiu-Jitsu, it includes joint locks, throws, and grappling techniques to control or subdue an opponent.

• **Forms (Kata):** Practitioners learn a series of pre-arranged movements, called forms or katas, which help develop muscle memory, balance, and coordination.

• **Self-Defense:** Practical self-defense techniques are a core component, teaching students how to respond to real-world threats and attacks.

Training and Philosophy:

Shaolin Kempo Karate emphasizes discipline, respect, and continuous improvement. Training typically involves a combination of:

1. **Physical Conditioning:** Building strength, flexibility, and endurance.

2. **Technique Practice:** Repetition of strikes, blocks, and forms to develop precision and power.

3. **Sparring:** Controlled practice with a partner to apply techniques in a dynamic setting.

4. **Mental Focus:** Cultivating concentration, awareness, and a calm mind under pressure.

Benefits:

Practicing Shaolin Kempo Karate offers numerous benefits, including:

1. **Self-Defense Skills:** Practical techniques for protecting oneself and others.

2. **Physical Fitness:** Improved strength, flexibility, and cardiovascular health.

3. **Mental Discipline:** Enhanced focus, patience, and resilience.

4. **Confidence:** Building self-esteem and a sense of accomplishment through mastery of skills.

Shaolin Kempo Karate is a versatile and effective martial art that provides a well-rounded approach to self-defense, fitness, and personal growth.

The Philosophy And Principles

Shaolin Kempo Karate is deeply rooted in the philosophies and principles that guide its practice. These concepts are essential for understanding the martial art's holistic approach, which goes beyond physical techniques to include mental and spiritual development.

1. Harmony and Balance: Shaolin Kempo Karate emphasizes the importance of harmony and balance, both within oneself and in interactions with others. This principle is reflected in the integration of various martial arts techniques, combining hard and soft movements to create a balanced and effective system.

2. Adaptability: A core principle is the ability to adapt to any situation. Practitioners are taught to be flexible in their responses, whether dealing with an opponent's attack or navigating life's challenges. This adaptability is cultivated through diverse training, which includes striking, grappling, and joint locks.

3. Respect and Humility: Respect for oneself, others, and the martial art itself is fundamental. Students are encouraged to practice humility, recognizing that there is always more to learn and that mastery is a continuous journey. This attitude fosters a positive training environment and personal growth.

4. Discipline and Self-Control: Shaolin Kempo Karate demands high levels of discipline and self-control. Practitioners must dedicate themselves to regular training, pushing through physical and mental barriers. This discipline extends beyond the dojo, influencing behavior and decision-making in daily life.

5. Perseverance: The path to proficiency in Shaolin Kempo Karate is challenging, requiring perseverance and resilience. Students learn to overcome obstacles, persist through difficulties, and remain committed to their goals. This tenacity is a crucial aspect of both martial arts training and personal development.

6. Mindfulness and Awareness: Mindfulness, or being fully present in the moment, is crucial in both practice and application. Practitioners develop acute awareness of their surroundings, their own movements, and their opponent's actions. This heightened state of awareness enhances reaction times and decision-making.

7. Self-Improvement: Continuous self-improvement is a key principle. Students are encouraged to constantly refine their techniques, expand their knowledge, and strive for personal betterment. This lifelong journey of growth is at the heart of Shaolin Kempo Karate.

8. Compassion and Benevolence: Despite its combat nature, Shaolin Kempo Karate promotes compassion and benevolence. Practitioners are taught to use their skills responsibly, avoiding unnecessary violence and seeking peaceful resolutions whenever possible. This principle underscores the martial art's ethical foundation.

9. Mental and Physical Unity: Shaolin Kempo Karate fosters the integration of mind and body. Techniques are not just physical movements but are driven by mental intent and focus. This unity enhances the effectiveness of techniques and contributes to overall well-being.

10. Wisdom and Knowledge: The pursuit of wisdom and knowledge is encouraged, both within the martial arts context and in broader life experiences. Understanding the principles behind techniques, learning from various sources, and applying martial arts philosophy to everyday life are vital aspects of Shaolin Kempo Karate.

The philosophy and principles of Shaolin Kempo Karate provide a comprehensive framework that guides practitioners in their training and personal development. By embracing these concepts, students not only become skilled martial artists but also develop the character, discipline, and mindset necessary for leading a balanced and fulfilling life.

CHAPTER 1: BASIC TECHNIQUES
Stances

In Shaolin Kempo Karate, stances form the foundation of movement and technique execution. They are essential for maintaining balance, generating power, and transitioning between strikes, blocks, and other maneuvers. Here are some of the fundamental stances in Shaolin Kempo Karate:

1. Horse Stance (Kiba Dachi):

• **Description:** The feet are positioned wider than shoulder-width apart, with the toes pointing slightly outward. The knees are bent deeply, and the hips are lowered to create a stable, grounded position.

• **Purpose:** This stance builds leg strength and stability. It is often used in training to develop endurance and is the starting point for many techniques.

2. Front Stance (Zenkutsu Dachi):

• **Description:** One foot is placed forward with the knee bent, while the back leg is straight. The front foot points forward, and the back foot is angled outward slightly. The weight is distributed primarily on the front leg.

• **Purpose:** The front stance provides a strong base for delivering powerful strikes and moving forward. It enhances stability and forward momentum.

3. Back Stance (Kokutsu Dachi):

• **Description:** The feet are positioned similarly to the front stance, but the majority of the weight is on the back leg. The front foot points forward, and the back foot is perpendicular to the front foot.

• **Purpose:** The back stance is used for defensive movements, allowing quick shifts backward and to the side while maintaining balance.

4. Cat Stance (Neko Ashi Dachi):

• **Description:** The majority of the weight is on the back leg, with the front foot lightly touching the ground, ready to move. The back leg is bent, and the front foot is positioned close to the back foot, with the heel slightly raised.

• **Purpose:** The cat stance is used for quick, agile movements and transitions. It allows for rapid changes in direction and quick strikes or blocks.

5. Cross Stance (Kosa Dachi):

• **Description:** One leg crosses behind or in front of the other, with both knees bent. The feet are positioned closely together, with the weight distributed evenly.

• **Purpose:** The cross stance is used for evasion and transitioning between other stances. It can also be employed in certain striking techniques.

6. Bow Stance (Gong Bu):

• **Description:** Similar to the front stance but with a deeper bend in the front knee and a lower overall posture. The back leg remains straight, and the front foot points forward.

• **Purpose:** The bow stance provides a stable base for powerful forward strikes and is commonly used in forms (katas).

7. Ready Stance (Yoi Dachi):

• **Description:** Feet are shoulder-width apart, with the knees slightly bent. The body is relaxed but ready to move in any direction.

• **Purpose:** The ready stance is a neutral position used to prepare for action. It allows for quick transitions into offensive or defensive movements.

8. Natural Stance (Shizentai):

• **Description:** The feet are positioned naturally, about shoulder-width apart, with the knees slightly bent and the body relaxed.

• **Purpose:** This stance is often used in beginning and ending forms, as well as in casual practice. It promotes relaxation and readiness.

9. Dragon Stance (Long Xiang Bu):

• **Description:** The front leg is bent, and the back leg is extended behind with the ball of the foot touching the ground. The upper body leans slightly forward.

• **Purpose:** The dragon stance is used for low, sweeping movements and transitions. It combines stability with fluidity.

10. Crane Stance (Tsuru Ashi Dachi):

• **Description:** One leg is raised, with the foot touching the inside of the opposite knee. The standing leg is slightly bent.

• **Purpose:** The crane stance is used for balance training and is often incorporated into forms for kicks and evasive maneuvers.

Stances are a crucial aspect of Shaolin Kempo Karate, forming the basis for effective movement and technique execution. Mastering these stances enhances balance, power, and agility, enabling practitioners to perform techniques with precision and confidence. Regular practice and mindful attention to stances are essential for developing a strong foundation in Shaolin Kempo Karate.

Footwork

Footwork in Shaolin Kempo Karate is essential for effective movement, allowing practitioners to position themselves advantageously, maintain balance, generate power, and execute techniques with precision. Here are some fundamental footwork techniques used in Shaolin Kempo Karate:

1. Step and Slide:

• **Description:** The lead foot steps forward or backward, and the rear foot follows to maintain stance and balance.

• **Purpose:** This movement is used to advance or retreat while maintaining a stable stance and readiness for strikes or blocks.

2. Shuffle Step:

• **Description:** Both feet move together, with the lead foot stepping forward or backward, and the rear foot quickly following.

• **Purpose:** The shuffle step is used for quick, short movements to adjust position without losing balance or opening up defenses.

3. Pivot:

• **Description:** The body rotates on the ball of one foot, while the other foot turns to change direction.

• **Purpose:** Pivoting allows for quick changes in direction, helping to evade attacks or reposition for a counterattack.

4. Crossover Step:

• **Description:** One foot crosses over the other, either in front or behind, to change direction or angle.

• **Purpose:** This step is used to create angles for attacks or to evade an opponent's line of attack.

5. Switch Step:

• **Description:** The lead and rear feet quickly switch positions.

• **Purpose:** The switch step is used to confuse an opponent, change stances, or quickly transition between offensive and defensive movements.

6. Triangle Step:

• **Description:** Movement follows a triangular pattern, with steps taken to the sides and forward or backward.

• **Purpose:** This step is used to create angles, improve positioning, and enhance evasive maneuvers.

7. Side Step (Lateral Movement):

• **Description:** The feet move sideways, maintaining the stance while shifting the body to the left or right.

• **Purpose:** Side stepping is used to evade attacks, create angles for counterattacks, and adjust positioning without moving forward or backward.

8. Circular Step:

• **Description:** The practitioner steps in a circular motion around the opponent.

• **Purpose:** Circular stepping helps to evade linear attacks and position oneself advantageously for strikes or grappling.

9. Backward Step:

• **Description:** The rear foot steps back, followed by the lead foot.

• **Purpose:** The backward step is used to create distance from an opponent's attack, preparing for a counter or a defensive maneuver.

10. Forward Step:

• **Description:** The lead foot steps forward, followed by the rear foot.

- **Purpose:** This step is used to close the distance to an opponent, enabling strikes, grappling, or other offensive techniques.

Application in Training

Footwork drills are a crucial part of Shaolin Kempo Karate training. These drills help students develop agility, speed, and precision. Common exercises include:

- **Shadow Boxing:** Practicing footwork and techniques against an imaginary opponent.

- **Partner Drills:** Working with a partner to practice footwork in response to attacks and movements.

- **Forms (Kata):** Performing forms that incorporate various footwork patterns to build muscle memory and fluidity.

Importance of Footwork

Good footwork is vital for several reasons:

• **Balance:** Proper footwork helps maintain balance during movements and techniques.

• **Power Generation:** Effective footwork positions the body to generate maximum power for strikes and blocks.

• **Evasion:** Quick and precise footwork allows for effective evasion of attacks.

• **Positioning:** Footwork helps achieve optimal positioning for both offensive and defensive maneuvers.

Mastering footwork in Shaolin Kempo Karate is essential for becoming a proficient martial artist. It enhances balance, agility, and the ability to execute techniques effectively. Consistent practice and mindful attention to footwork will significantly improve overall performance and effectiveness in both training and real-world self-defense situations.

Basic Blocks

In Shaolin Kempo Karate, basic blocks are essential techniques used to defend against incoming attacks. These blocks help protect vital areas of the body and create openings for counterattacks. Here are some of the fundamental blocks in Shaolin Kempo Karate:

1. High Block (Jodan Uke):

• **Description:** The arm rises to deflect an incoming attack aimed at the head or upper body. The blocking arm is bent at the elbow, and the forearm is angled upward.

• **Purpose:** This block is used to protect the head and upper body from high strikes, such as punches or kicks.

2. Middle Block (Chudan Uke):

• **Description:** The arm moves outward from the center of the body to deflect a mid-level attack. The forearm is angled to intercept strikes aimed at the torso.

• **Purpose:** This block is used to defend against punches or kicks directed at the midsection.

3. Low Block (Gedan Barai):

• **Description:** The arm sweeps downward to deflect an attack aimed at the lower body. The forearm is angled to redirect the strike away from the legs or groin.

• **Purpose:** This block is used to protect the lower body from kicks or other low attacks.

4. Inside Block (Uchi Uke)

• **Description:** The arm moves from the outside toward the centerline of the body to intercept an incoming attack. The forearm is angled inward.

• **Purpose:** This block is used to deflect strikes coming from the side, such as hooks or roundhouse punches.

5. Outside Block (Soto Uke):

• **Description:** The arm moves from the centerline outward to deflect an attack. The forearm is angled outward.

• **Purpose:** This block is used to protect against linear strikes coming directly at the body, such as jabs or straight punches.

6. Palm Block (Shotei Uke):

• **Description:** The open hand moves to intercept and deflect an attack. The palm faces outward, and the fingers are extended.

• **Purpose:** This block is used to redirect attacks with the palm, providing a larger surface area for deflection.

7. Cross Block (Juji Uke):

• **Description:** Both arms cross in front of the body to create an "X" shape, intercepting an incoming attack.

• **Purpose:** This block is used for strong, two-handed defense against powerful strikes or to trap an opponent's limb.

8. Rising Block (Age Uke):

• **Description:** The arm moves upward with the palm facing the opponent, intercepting high strikes.

• **Purpose:** Similar to the high block, this block is used to protect the head from downward strikes.

9. Knife-Hand Block (Shuto Uke):

• **Description:** The arm moves with an open hand, using the edge of the hand (knife-hand) to deflect an attack.

• **Purpose:** This block is used to intercept strikes with precision and is often followed by a counterattack using the knife-hand.

10. Hooking Block (Kake Uke):

• **Description:** The arm hooks inward to catch and redirect an incoming attack.

Purpose: This block is used to trap or control an opponent's limb, setting up for a counterattack.

Application in Training:

Blocks are practiced through various drills and forms to develop speed, accuracy, and effectiveness. Common training methods include:

• **Basic Drills:** Repetition of each block to build muscle memory and refine technique.

• **Partner Drills:** Practicing blocks with a partner who simulates attacks, helping to develop timing and reaction speed.

• **Forms (Kata):** Incorporating blocks into forms to understand their application in combination with other techniques.

Importance of Proper Blocking:

Effective blocking is crucial for several reasons:

• **Protection:** Blocks shield vital areas of the body from injury.

• **Control:** Proper blocking can disrupt an opponent's attack and create opportunities for counterattacks.

• **Confidence:** Mastery of blocking techniques enhances overall confidence in one's defensive capabilities.

Mastering basic blocks in Shaolin Kempo Karate is fundamental to becoming an effective martial artist. These techniques provide essential protection and form the foundation for more advanced defensive and offensive maneuvers. Consistent practice and mindful application of blocks will significantly improve overall martial arts proficiency and self-defense skills.

Basic Strikes

In Shaolin Kempo Karate, basic strikes are fundamental techniques used for offense, counterattacks, and self-defense. Mastering these strikes involves understanding proper form, targeting, and power generation. Here are some of the essential strikes in Shaolin Kempo Karate:

1. Jab (Kizami Zuki):

• **Description:** A quick, straight punch thrown with the lead hand.

• **Purpose:** Used to probe, distract, or set up for more powerful strikes. It targets the opponent's head or torso.

2. Cross (Gyaku Zuki):

• **Description:** A powerful, straight punch thrown with the rear hand, rotating the hips and shoulders to generate force.

• **Purpose:** This punch delivers significant power and is aimed at the opponent's head or torso.

3. Front Kick (Mae Geri);

• **Description:** A straightforward kick delivered with the ball of the foot or the heel, targeting the opponent's midsection or head.

• **Purpose:** Used to keep an opponent at a distance or deliver a powerful blow to the torso or head.

4. Roundhouse Kick (Mawashi Geri):

• **Description:** A circular kick delivered with the instep or the ball of the foot, aimed at the opponent's ribs, head, or legs.

• **Purpose:** This kick is effective for striking from the side, with significant power and reach.

5. Side Kick (Yoko Geri):

• **Description:** A powerful kick delivered to the side, using the heel or the edge of the foot, targeting the opponent's midsection or head.

• **Purpose:** This kick is used for its reach and power, often to break through an opponent's guard.

6. Hook Punch (Kagi Zuki):

• **Description:** A punch delivered in a hooking motion, with the fist traveling horizontally to strike the opponent's jaw or body.

• **Purpose:** Effective for targeting the sides of an opponent's head or body, often following a jab or cross.

7. Uppercut (Age Zuki):

• **Description:** An upward punch delivered with a bent elbow, aiming for the opponent's chin or solar plexus.

• **Purpose:** This punch is useful for close-range attacks, particularly when targeting the chin or midsection.

8. Back Fist Strike (Uraken Uchi):

• **Description:** A quick strike delivered with the back of the fist, often targeting the face or temple.

• **Purpose:** This strike is fast and can catch an opponent off guard, typically used in close-range combat.

9. Elbow Strike (Empi Uchi):

• **Description:** A strike using the elbow, delivered in various directions (upward, downward, sideways) to target the opponent's head or body.

• **Purpose:** Elbow strikes are powerful and effective at close range, useful for infighting or breaking through an opponent's guard.

10. Palm Heel Strike (Shotei Uchi):

• **Description:** A strike delivered with the base of the palm, targeting the opponent's chin, nose, or solar plexus.

• **Purpose:** This strike minimizes the risk of injury to the hand and is effective for pushing or driving through an opponent.

11. Knife-Hand Strike (Shuto Uchi):

• **Description:** A strike using the edge of the open hand, targeting the neck, temple, or other vulnerable areas.

• **Purpose:** Known for its precision and power, the knife-hand strike can be used to disable an opponent effectively.

12. Knee Strike (Hiza Geri):

• **Description:** A strike using the knee, often aimed at the opponent's midsection, groin, or head.

• **Purpose:** Knee strikes are powerful close-range attacks, useful for inflicting significant damage.

Application in Training

Strikes are practiced through various drills to develop speed, accuracy, and power. Common training methods include:

• **Pad Work:** Practicing strikes against pads or focus mitts to develop power and precision.

• **Shadow Boxing:** Rehearsing strikes in the air to perfect form and technique.

• **Bag Work:** Using heavy bags to build power and endurance.

• **Partner Drills:** Working with a partner to practice strikes and combinations in a controlled environment.

Importance of Proper Striking Technique

Effective striking is crucial for several reasons:

• **Power:** Proper technique maximizes the power of each strike.

• **Speed:** Efficient movement ensures strikes are delivered quickly.

• **Accuracy:** Correct form improves precision, increasing the likelihood of hitting intended targets.

• **Safety:** Proper technique reduces the risk of self-injury during training and application.

Mastering basic strikes in Shaolin Kempo Karate is essential for becoming a proficient martial artist. These techniques provide the foundation for offensive and counter-offensive maneuvers. Regular practice and mindful attention to form and application will significantly enhance striking effectiveness and overall martial arts proficiency.

CHAPTER 2: INTERMEDIATE TECHNIQUES

Advanced Stances

Advanced stances in Shaolin Kempo Karate build upon the fundamental stances, incorporating more complex positioning and transitions.

These stances enhance balance, power generation, and strategic movement, allowing practitioners to perform advanced techniques effectively. Here are some of the advanced stances in Shaolin Kempo Karate:

1. Crane Stance (Tsuru Ashi Dachi):

• **Description:** One leg is raised with the foot touching the inside of the opposite knee, and the standing leg is slightly bent. The hands are often positioned for a strike or block.

- **Purpose:** This stance develops balance and stability and is used to execute quick kicks or evasive maneuvers.

2. Dragon Stance (Long Xiang Bu):

- **Description:** The front leg is bent deeply, and the back leg is extended behind with the ball of the foot touching the ground. The upper body leans slightly forward.

- **Purpose:** This stance is used for low, sweeping movements and transitions, combining stability with fluidity.

3. Low Stance (Shiko Dachi):

- **Description:** Similar to the horse stance but with a wider and lower position, with the feet pointing outward and knees deeply bent.

• **Purpose:** This stance builds leg strength and stability and is used for powerful, grounded techniques.

4. X-Stance (Kosa Dachi):

• **Description:** One leg crosses behind or in front of the other, and both knees are bent. The feet are positioned closely together.

• **Purpose:** This stance is used for evasion and transitioning between other stances, offering quick changes in direction.

5. Cat Stance (Neko Ashi Dachi):

• **Description:** The majority of the weight is on the back leg, with the front foot lightly touching the ground and the heel slightly raised.

• **Purpose:** This stance allows for quick, agile movements and transitions, facilitating rapid strikes or blocks.

6. Cross-legged Stance (Kake Dachi):

• **Description:** One leg crosses tightly in front of the other, with the knees bent and the body slightly lowered.

• **Purpose:** This stance is used for close-range techniques and evasion, allowing quick directional changes.

7. Back Stance (Kokutsu Dachi):

• **Description:** The weight is mostly on the back leg, with the front foot pointing forward and the back foot perpendicular.

• **Purpose:** This defensive stance allows for quick shifts backward and lateral movements, preparing for counterattacks.

8. Forward Leaning Stance (Zenkutsu Dachi):

• **Description:** The front leg is bent deeply, and the back leg is straight. The body leans forward, distributing weight evenly.

• **Purpose:** This stance provides a strong base for powerful forward strikes and is commonly used in offensive techniques.

9. Half-moon Stance (Hangetsu Dachi):

• **Description:** The feet are placed shoulder-width apart, with the knees slightly bent and the toes pointing inward. The stance forms a half-moon shape.

• **Purpose:** This stance is used for stability and balance, allowing for smooth transitions and power generation in circular movements.

10. **One-legged Stance (Ippon Ashi Dachi)**

Description: One leg is raised, and the body weight is balanced on the standing leg. The raised leg can be positioned in various ways, such as preparing for a kick.

Purpose: This stance develops balance and control, and is used for executing kicks or preparing for advanced techniques.

Application in Training

Advanced stances are practiced through various drills and forms to develop mastery. Common training methods include:

Kata (Forms): Practicing advanced stances within kata to understand their application in combination with techniques.

Partner Drills: Working with a partner to practice transitions and movements between advanced stances.

Balance Exercises: Performing exercises to enhance stability and control in advanced stances.

Sparring: Applying advanced stances in sparring sessions to develop practical usage and adaptability.

Importance of Advanced Stances

Mastering advanced stances is crucial for several reasons:

Stability: Advanced stances provide a stable base for executing complex techniques.

Power Generation: Proper stance allows for maximum power generation in strikes and blocks.

Balance: Advanced stances enhance balance, enabling smooth transitions and fluid movements.

Strategic Positioning: These stances offer strategic advantages in positioning and movement, aiding both offense and defense.

Conclusion

Advanced stances in Shaolin Kempo Karate build on the basics, offering greater complexity and strategic options. Mastering these stances enhances a practitioner's overall martial arts proficiency, providing the foundation for advanced techniques and effective self-defense. Consistent practice and mindful application of these stances will significantly improve balance, stability, and power in martial arts performance.

Combination Techniques

Combination techniques in Shaolin Kempo Karate involve integrating multiple strikes, blocks, and movements into fluid sequences. These combinations are designed to create openings, exploit weaknesses, and deliver powerful attacks while maintaining defense. Here are some fundamental combination techniques in Shaolin Kempo Karate:

1. Jab-Cross-Hook Combination:

• **Description:** Start with a quick jab (lead hand), followed by a powerful cross (rear hand), and finish with a hook punch (lead hand).

• **Purpose:** This combination is used to disrupt the opponent's guard, deliver powerful strikes, and target different angles.

2. Front Kick-Punch Combination:

• **Description:** Execute a front kick (lead leg) to the opponent's midsection or head, immediately followed by a cross punch (rear hand).

• **Purpose:** The kick creates distance or off-balances the opponent, while the punch capitalizes on the opening.

3. Low Block-Roundhouse Kick:

• **Description:** Start with a low block to deflect an incoming low attack, followed by a roundhouse kick (rear leg) aimed at the opponent's midsection or head.

• **Purpose:** This combination is effective for defending against low attacks and countering with a powerful strike.

4. Side Kick-Back Fist Combination:

• **Description:** Deliver a side kick (rear leg) to the opponent's midsection, followed by a back fist strike (lead hand) to the head.

- **Purpose:** The side kick creates distance and off-balances the opponent, while the back fist targets a high opening.

5. Inside Block-Elbow Strike:

- **Description:** Perform an inside block to deflect an incoming attack, followed by an elbow strike (same arm) to the opponent's head or body.

- **Purpose:** This combination is used for close-range defense and counterattacking with a powerful, compact strike.

6. Jab-Front Kick-Cross:

- **Description:** Begin with a quick jab to disrupt the opponent's guard, follow with a front kick to the midsection, and finish with a cross punch.

• **Purpose:** The jab sets up the kick, and the kick creates an opening for the powerful cross punch.

7. Hook Punch-Uppercut Combination:

• **Description:** Deliver a hook punch (lead hand) to the opponent's head or body, immediately followed by an uppercut (rear hand) to the chin or solar plexus.

• **Purpose:** This combination targets multiple angles, making it difficult for the opponent to defend effectively.

8. Palm Heel Strike-Knee Strike:

• **Description:** Execute a palm heel strike to the opponent's chin or nose, followed by a knee strike to the midsection or groin.

- **Purpose:** The palm heel strike off-balances the opponent, creating an opening for the powerful knee strike.

9. Knife-Hand Block-Ridge Hand Strike:

- **Description:** Perform a knife-hand block to deflect an incoming strike, followed by a ridge hand strike (same arm) to the opponent's neck or temple.

- **Purpose:** This combination uses the same arm for defense and counterattack, allowing for a quick and fluid response.

10. Sweep-Takedown Combination:

- **Description:** Use a sweeping motion (rear leg) to off-balance the opponent, followed by a takedown technique to bring them to the ground.

• **Purpose:** This combination is effective for transitioning from standing strikes to ground control.

Application in Training

Combination techniques are practiced through various drills to develop fluidity, timing, and effectiveness. Common training methods include:

• **Pad Work:** Practicing combinations against pads or focus mitts to develop power and precision.

• **Shadow Boxing:** Rehearsing combinations in the air to perfect form and technique.

• **Partner Drills:** Working with a partner to practice combinations in a controlled environment, focusing on timing and accuracy.

- **Sparring:** Applying combinations in sparring sessions to develop practical usage and adaptability.

Importance of Combination Techniques

Mastering combination techniques is crucial for several reasons:

- **Fluidity:** Combos help practitioners move seamlessly between techniques, maintaining offensive pressure.

- **Adaptability:** Combinations train practitioners to adapt to an opponent's movements and create openings.

- **Power Generation:** Fluid transitions between techniques enhance power generation and effectiveness.

• **Defense and Offense:** Combining strikes and blocks ensures balanced offense and defense, reducing vulnerability.

Combination techniques in Shaolin Kempo Karate integrate multiple strikes, blocks, and movements into cohesive sequences, enhancing overall effectiveness. Regular practice of these combinations develops fluidity, power, and strategic adaptability, crucial for both training and real-world self-defense.

Defense Against Grabs

Defense against grabs in Shaolin Kempo Karate focuses on techniques that allow practitioners to escape, counterattack, and control the situation when an opponent attempts to grab them. These techniques involve leveraging body mechanics, striking vulnerable areas, and using joint locks or throws to neutralize the threat. Here are some essential defense techniques against grabs:

1. Wrist Grab Defense

Single-Hand Wrist Grab:

Technique:

- **Escape:** Rotate your wrist towards the opponent's thumb, the weakest part of their grip, and pull your hand free.

• **Counter:** Follow up with a strike, such as a palm heel to the face or a knee strike to the midsection.

• **Purpose:** This technique uses leverage to break the grip and immediately transitions to an offensive move.

Double-Hand Wrist Grab

Technique:

• **Escape:** Use your free hand to strike the opponent's hand or face, then twist your wrist to break free.

• **Counter:** Follow up with an elbow strike to the face or a front kick to the midsection.

• **Purpose:** Striking the opponent distracts them, making it easier to break the grip and counterattack.

2. Clothing Grab Defense

Lapel Grab

Technique:

• **Escape:** Trap the opponent's grabbing hand with one of your hands, then use your other hand to strike the opponent's face or throat.

• **Counter:** Apply a wrist lock or armbar to control the opponent, or execute a knee strike to the groin.

• **Purpose:** This technique combines controlling the grab with a powerful strike to disable the opponent.

Shoulder Grab

Technique:

• **Escape:** Turn your body towards the grabbing hand while striking the opponent's wrist or forearm to break the grip.

• **Counter:** Follow up with a back fist strike to the face or an elbow strike to the ribs.

• **Purpose:** The turning motion helps to weaken the grip, and the counterstrike capitalizes on the opening.

3. Bear Hug Defense

Bear Hug from the Front (Arms Free)

Technique:

• **Escape:** Use your hands to push against the opponent's hips or lower body, creating space.

• **Counter:** Follow up with a knee strike to the groin or an upward elbow strike to the chin.

• **Purpose:** Creating space weakens the grip and allows for powerful counterattacks.

Bear Hug from the Front (Arms Pinned)

Technique:

• **Escape:** Use your hips to shift to one side, creating space for your hands. Use your hands to push against the opponent's hips.

• **Counter:** Follow up with a headbutt to the opponent's face or a knee strike to the groin.

• **Purpose:** The hip movement creates space, enabling effective counterattacks.

Bear Hug from Behind (Arms Free)

Technique:

• **Escape:** Use your elbows to strike the opponent's ribs or head.

• **Counter:** Follow up with a stomp to the opponent's foot or a backward headbutt.

• **Purpose:** Striking with the elbows weakens the grip, allowing for effective counterattacks.

Bear Hug from Behind (Arms Pinned)

Technique:

• **Escape:** Drop your weight and shift to one side to create space. Use your hands to push against the opponent's hips.

* **Counter:** Follow up with a backward headbutt or a heel stomp to the opponent's foot.

* **Purpose:** Dropping your weight creates space and makes it easier to counterattack.

4. Choke Hold Defense

Front Choke

Technique:

* **Escape:** Use both hands to strike the opponent's arms inward, breaking their grip.

* **Counter:** Follow up with a palm heel strike to the opponent's face or a knee strike to the midsection.

* **Purpose:** Striking the arms breaks the choke, allowing for immediate counterattacks.

Rear Choke

Technique:

• **Escape:** Tuck your chin to protect your throat, use your hands to pull down on the opponent's forearm.

• **Counter:** Follow up with a backward headbutt or an elbow strike to the opponent's ribs.

• **Purpose:** Protecting the throat and pulling down on the arm weakens the choke, enabling effective counterattacks.

Application in Training

• Defense against grabs is practiced through various drills to develop speed, precision, and effectiveness. Common training methods include:

• **Partner Drills:** Practicing defense techniques with a partner simulating grabs to develop timing and accuracy.

• **Self-Defense Scenarios:** Simulating real-life situations to practice applying techniques under pressure.

• **Technique Drills:** Repetitively practicing specific defenses to build muscle memory and confidence.

• **Sparring:** Applying grab defenses in controlled sparring sessions to develop practical usage and adaptability.

Importance of Defense Against Grabs

Mastering defense against grabs is crucial for several reasons:

• **Safety:** Effective techniques ensure personal safety in real-life self-defense situations.

• **Confidence:** Confidence in handling grabs reduces fear and hesitation in confrontations.

• **Control:** Proper techniques allow for control over the situation, preventing escalation.

• **Adaptability:** Training in various scenarios enhances adaptability and quick thinking in unexpected situations.

Defense against grabs in Shaolin Kempo Karate involves leveraging body mechanics, striking, and joint manipulation to neutralize threats. Regular practice of these techniques develops the necessary skills to handle various grabbing attacks effectively, enhancing overall self-defense capabilities.

CHAPTER 3: FORMS (KATA)
Importance Of Forms In Shaolin Kempo Karate

Forms, or kata, play a vital role in Shaolin Kempo Karate, serving as foundational exercises that encompass a wide range of techniques, movements, and principles. They are structured sequences of movements that combine stances, strikes, blocks, and footwork, embodying the essence of martial arts practice. Here are some of the key reasons why forms are important in Shaolin Kempo Karate:

1. Technique Mastery:

• **Repetition and Refinement:** Forms provide practitioners with the opportunity to practice and refine their techniques repetitively. This repetition helps in developing muscle memory and improving precision in movements.

• **Focus on Detail:** Practicing forms allows students to focus on the details of each technique, ensuring proper form, balance, and alignment.

2. Physical Conditioning:

• **Strength and Flexibility:** Forms involve various movements that help build strength, flexibility, and endurance. Regular practice improves overall physical fitness, which is essential for effective martial arts performance.

• **Coordination and Balance:** The dynamic movements in forms enhance coordination and balance, crucial attributes for executing techniques effectively in combat scenarios.

3. Mental Discipline:

• **Focus and Concentration:** Practicing forms requires mental focus and concentration, helping students develop discipline and mindfulness. This mental training is beneficial both in martial arts and daily life.

• **Memory Development:** Learning and memorizing forms enhances cognitive abilities, improving memory retention and mental acuity.

4. Understanding Principles:

• **Application of Techniques:** Forms teach practitioners how to apply various techniques in a sequence, illustrating concepts such as timing, distance, and flow. This understanding is essential for effective combat application.

• **Combining Techniques:** Forms integrate different strikes, blocks, and movements, allowing students to see how techniques work together in a coherent manner, enhancing strategic thinking in combat.

5. Self-Defense Skills:

• **Practical Application:** Many forms incorporate self-defense techniques, providing a foundation for applying these skills in real-life situations. Practicing forms helps students recognize opportunities for counters and defensive maneuvers.

• **Scenario Training:** Forms simulate various combat scenarios, helping students prepare for potential encounters and develop their ability to respond effectively under pressure.

6. Cultural and Philosophical Significance:

• **Tradition and Heritage:** Forms are an essential aspect of martial arts culture, preserving techniques and philosophies passed down through generations. They connect practitioners to the history and traditions of their martial art.

• **Personal Growth:** Practicing forms encourages self-reflection and personal development, fostering qualities such as humility, respect, and perseverance, which are essential values in martial arts.

7. Competition Preparation:

• **Tournament Readiness:** Forms are often a part of competitions, allowing practitioners to showcase their skills. Regular practice prepares students for performance in front of judges and peers, improving confidence and poise.

• **Skill Evaluation:** Forms provide a means of evaluating a practitioner's skill level, allowing instructors to assess progress and areas for improvement.

Forms are an integral part of Shaolin Kempo Karate, offering a structured approach to mastering techniques, improving physical fitness, and developing mental discipline. They serve as a bridge between traditional martial arts and practical application, emphasizing the importance of both technique and philosophy. Regular practice of forms not only enhances martial arts skills but also contributes to personal growth and self-improvement, making them essential for any serious student of Shaolin Kempo Karate.

Beginner Forms

Beginner forms in Shaolin Kempo Karate are designed to introduce new practitioners to the foundational movements, stances, and techniques of the martial art. These forms emphasize proper technique, body mechanics, and basic principles, allowing students to build a solid foundation for further advancement. Here are some common beginner forms:

1. Heian Shodan (Peaceful Mind First Level)

• **Description:** This is often one of the first forms taught to beginners. It consists of basic stances, blocks, and punches, emphasizing proper footwork and transitions.

Key Techniques:

1.   Front Stance (Zenkutsu Dachi)

2.   Low Block (Gedan Barai)

3.   Middle Punch (Chudan Tsuki)

Focus: Developing balance, coordination, and understanding of basic strikes and blocks.

2. Heian Nidan (Peaceful Mind Second Level)

• **Description:** This form builds upon the skills learned in Heian Shodan, introducing new techniques and combinations.

Key Techniques:

1.   Side Stance (Kiba Dachi)

2.   High Block (Jodan Uke)

3.   Front Kick (Mae Geri)

Focus: Enhancing footwork, introducing kicks, and further refining blocking techniques.

3. Heian Sandan (Peaceful Mind Third Level)

• **Description:** This form continues to build on previous forms, incorporating more advanced techniques and transitions.

Key Techniques:

1. Back Stance (Kokutsu Dachi)
2. Downward Block (Gedan Uke)
3. Hook Punch (Kage Tsuki)

• **Focus:** Developing fluid transitions between stances and techniques, improving coordination.

4. Kihon Kata (Basic Form):

• **Description:** A simplified form focusing solely on basic techniques without complex transitions. This form is excellent for beginners to practice foundational skills.

Key Techniques:

1. Basic Stances (Zenkutsu, Kiba, Kokutsu Dachi)
2. Basic Strikes (Jab, Cross, Front Kick)

Focus: Reinforcing foundational movements and techniques, promoting muscle memory.

5. Tai Chi Form (Beginner Level):

• **Description:** While not exclusive to Kempo, some schools incorporate a basic Tai Chi form to help beginners with relaxation, balance, and fluid movement.

Key Techniques:

1. Slow, controlled movements
2. Focus on breathing and flow

Focus: Promoting relaxation, balance, and mental focus, providing a contrast to more dynamic techniques.

6. Basic Self-Defense Techniques:

• **Description:** In addition to traditional forms, beginners often practice basic self-defense techniques that incorporate elements of forms.

Key Techniques:

1. Wrist escapes
2. Basic blocking and countering against grabs

Focus: Understanding practical applications of techniques learned in forms and enhancing confidence in self-defense scenarios.

Application in Training

• **Repetitive Practice:** Beginners should practice these forms repeatedly to build muscle memory and improve technique.

• **Guided Instruction:** Working with instructors or using instructional videos can help ensure proper form and execution.

• **Partner Drills:** Practicing forms with partners allows students to apply techniques in simulated scenarios, enhancing understanding and adaptability.

<u>**Importance of Beginner Forms**</u>

• **Foundation Building:** Beginner forms establish the essential skills necessary for more advanced techniques and forms.

• **Confidence Development:** Mastering basic forms instills confidence in new practitioners as they see their skills improve.

• **Discipline and Focus:** Practicing forms cultivates mental discipline, focus, and attention to detail, which are vital in martial arts training.

Beginner forms in Shaolin Kempo Karate are crucial for introducing new practitioners to the essential techniques, stances, and movements of the martial art. Through consistent practice and dedication, students can develop a strong foundation that supports their journey in martial arts, enhancing their physical and mental capabilities.

Intermediate Forms

Intermediate forms in Shaolin Kempo Karate build upon the foundational techniques learned in beginner forms, introducing more complex movements, combinations, and strategies. These forms help practitioners refine their skills, improve their understanding of martial arts principles, and develop their ability to apply techniques in various scenarios. Here are some common intermediate forms:

1. Heian Yondan (Peaceful Mind Fourth Level)

• **Description:** This form introduces more advanced techniques and combinations, emphasizing fluidity and coordination between movements.

Key Techniques:

1. Back Stance (Kokutsu Dachi)
2. Side Block (Yoko Uke)
3. Back Fist Strike (Uraken)

Focus: Enhancing transitions between techniques and developing a deeper understanding of distance and timing.

2. Heian Godan (Peaceful Mind Fifth Level):

• **Description:** This form builds on the complexity of the previous Heian forms, incorporating more dynamic movements and techniques.

Key Techniques:

1. Cat Stance (Neko Ashi Dachi)
2. Jumping Front Kick (Tobi Mae Geri)
3. Knee Strike (Hiza Geri)

Focus: Developing agility and timing while combining different types of strikes and footwork.

3. Kanku Dai (Viewing the Sky):

• **Description:** Kanku Dai is a more advanced form that includes a wide variety of techniques, stances, and transitions. It is often introduced at the intermediate level.

Key Techniques:

- High Block (Jodan Uke)
- Roundhouse Kick (Mawashi Geri)
- Elbow Strike (Hiji Uchi)

Focus: Understanding the flow of techniques and practicing powerful strikes and defensive movements.

4. Gekisai Dai Ichi (Attack and Destroy First Level):

• **Description:** This form emphasizes practical self-defense applications and incorporates techniques that can be used in real-life scenarios.

Key Techniques:

1. Lunge Punch (Oi Tsuki)
2. Low Block (Gedan Barai)
3. Side Kick (Yoko Geri)

Focus: Integrating techniques into practical applications, emphasizing power and control.

5. Kihon Kata (Intermediate Level):

• **Description:** This form expands on the basic Kihon Kata by adding new techniques and combinations.

Key Techniques:

1. Combination Strikes (e.g., Jab-Cross-Hook)
2. Kicking Techniques (e.g., Front Kick, Side Kick)

Focus: Reinforcing the principles of timing and distance while applying combinations in a structured form.

6. Advanced Self-Defense Techniques:

• **Description:** In addition to traditional forms, intermediate students practice self-defense techniques that apply the principles learned in forms.

Key Techniques:

- Defenses against multiple attackers
- Joint locks and takedowns

Focus: Developing practical applications for techniques and enhancing confidence in self-defense scenarios.

Application in Training:

• **Partner Drills:** Practicing intermediate forms with partners allows for the application of techniques in dynamic situations, enhancing adaptability and responsiveness.

• **Shadow Training:** Solo practice of intermediate forms promotes muscle memory and focus on precision and technique.

• **Video Analysis:** Recording practice sessions can help identify areas for improvement and refine execution.

Importance of Intermediate Forms:

• **Skill Advancement:** Intermediate forms allow practitioners to progress beyond basics, developing a broader range of skills and techniques.

• **Confidence Building:** Mastery of intermediate forms enhances confidence and prepares students for more advanced techniques and forms.

• **Tactical Thinking:** Practicing these forms cultivates critical thinking and adaptability, essential for effective self-defense and sparring.

Intermediate forms in Shaolin Kempo Karate are crucial for expanding a practitioner's skill set, integrating more complex techniques, and fostering a deeper understanding of martial arts principles. Through dedicated practice, students develop confidence, precision, and adaptability, laying the groundwork for further advancement in their martial arts journey.

Advanced Forms

Advanced forms in Shaolin Kempo Karate are designed for practitioners who have mastered the foundational and intermediate techniques. These forms incorporate complex movements, combinations, and strategies that enhance a student's technical proficiency, physical conditioning, and mental focus. They serve as a bridge to high-level skills and competition. Here are some common advanced forms:

1. Kanku Sho (Small Viewing the Sky):

• **Description:** Kanku Sho is a shorter, more advanced form that emphasizes fluidity, rhythm, and the connection between movements. It serves as an introduction to more complex techniques and concepts.

Key Techniques:

1. Jumping Techniques (Tobi Geri)
2. Spinning Techniques (Mawashi Uchi)
3. Combination Strikes and Blocks

Focus: Mastering the flow of techniques and improving agility and balance through dynamic movements.

2. Gekisai Dai Ni (Attack and Destroy Second Level):

• **Description:** This form builds upon the principles established in Gekisai Dai Ichi, introducing more advanced techniques and combinations that emphasize practical application.

Key Techniques:

1. Crescent Kick (Mikazuki Geri)

2. Elbow and Knee Strikes

3. Advanced Blocking Techniques

Focus: Combining strikes, blocks, and evasive maneuvers to create effective self-defense applications.

3. Sochin (Stability):

• **Description:** Sochin is an advanced kata characterized by strong stances and powerful movements, emphasizing stability, control, and focus.

Key Techniques:

1. Sanchin Stance (Sanchin Dachi)

2. Powerful Strikes (e.g., Spear Hand)

3. Low and High Blocks

• **Focus:** Building inner strength, enhancing body mechanics, and practicing powerful techniques.

4. Tekki Shodan (Iron Horse First Level):

• **Description:** Tekki Shodan emphasizes lateral movements and powerful strikes from a horse stance, focusing on stability and precision.

Key Techniques:

1. Horse Stance (Kiba Dachi)
2. Side Punch (Yoko Tsuki)
3. Knees and Elbows

Focus: Strengthening lower body stability while developing precision in striking techniques.

5. Chinte (Rare Hands):

• **Description:** Chinte is a unique kata that incorporates unusual techniques and transitions, emphasizing creativity and adaptability in combat.

Key Techniques:

1. Specialized Strikes (e.g., Phoenix Eye Fist)
2. Throws and Takedowns
3. Unconventional Footwork

Focus: Encouraging improvisation and strategic thinking in various combat scenarios.

6. Advanced Self-Defense Techniques:

• **Description:** Advanced practitioners refine their self-defense skills, applying techniques learned in forms to real-life scenarios.

Key Techniques:

1. Defenses against multiple attackers
2. Complex joint locks and throws
3. Counterattack strategies

Focus: Developing practical applications of advanced techniques while enhancing confidence and situational awareness.

<u>Application in Training:</u>

• **Sparring Sessions:** Engaging in controlled sparring allows advanced practitioners to apply techniques from forms in dynamic situations, enhancing adaptability and reflexes.

• **Partner Drills:** Practicing advanced forms with partners helps solidify timing and execution in more realistic settings.

• **Performance Preparation:** Practicing forms for competitions enhances presentation skills and builds confidence in showcasing techniques.

Importance of Advanced Forms:

• **Skill Refinement:** Advanced forms help practitioners refine their techniques, emphasizing precision, speed, and power.

• **Creativity and Adaptability:** Practicing these forms encourages innovative thinking and adaptability in combat, essential for advanced practitioners.

• **Preparation for Mastery:** Mastering advanced forms prepares students for black belt testing and beyond, reinforcing the principles and techniques essential for high-level martial arts practice.

Advanced forms in Shaolin Kempo Karate are crucial for practitioners seeking to elevate their skills and understanding of martial arts. By incorporating complex movements and techniques, these forms enhance physical and mental capabilities, preparing students for higher levels of proficiency and mastery. Through dedicated practice, advanced practitioners cultivate confidence, precision, and adaptability, furthering their journey in martial arts.

CHAPTER 4: SPARRING
Introduction To Sparring

Sparring is a fundamental aspect of martial arts training, providing practitioners with the opportunity to apply techniques, develop timing, and enhance their overall combat skills in a controlled environment.

In Shaolin Kempo Karate, sparring is a crucial component that helps students transition from practicing forms and techniques to real-life applications. Here's an overview of sparring, its significance, and what practitioners can expect:

Sparring refers to practice fighting or controlled combat training between two martial artists. It can vary in intensity and rules, ranging from light contact drills focusing on technique to more intense, full-contact exchanges. In Shaolin Kempo

Karate, sparring can be categorized into different formats, including:

• **Controlled Sparring:** Practitioners focus on applying techniques without excessive force, emphasizing skill development and strategy.

• **Point Sparring:** A competitive format where participants score points for controlled strikes on specific targets, often using a referee to oversee the action.

• **Continuous Sparring:** Involves longer exchanges with an emphasis on maintaining fluidity and rhythm, allowing for more extended combinations of techniques.

Importance of Sparring in Martial Arts:

• **Practical Application:** Sparring allows students to practice techniques learned in forms and drills in a dynamic, unpredictable setting. It helps bridge the gap between theoretical knowledge and practical execution.

• **Timing and Distance Control:** Practicing with a partner teaches students to judge distances, improve timing, and learn when to engage or retreat based on their opponent's movements.

• **Improving Reflexes:** The unpredictable nature of sparring enhances a practitioner's reflexes and response time, vital skills for effective self-defense and competition.

• **Strategic Thinking:** Sparring requires practitioners to think critically and adapt their strategies in real-time, enhancing their ability to make quick decisions under pressure.

- **Building Confidence:** Regular sparring sessions help build confidence in one's abilities, allowing practitioners to feel more comfortable in applying their techniques in various situations.

- **Physical Conditioning:** Sparring is an excellent form of cardiovascular exercise, improving overall fitness levels, strength, and endurance, which are essential for effective martial arts performance.

Safety and Etiquette in Sparring:

- **Protective Gear:** Practitioners should wear appropriate protective gear, such as gloves, mouthguards, shin guards, and headgear, to minimize the risk of injury during sparring sessions.

- **Controlled Environment:** Sparring should be conducted in a safe, supervised environment where instructors can provide guidance and monitor for safety.

• **Respect and Sportsmanship:** Sparring partners should show respect for each other, maintain sportsmanship, and prioritize safety over winning. The goal is to learn and improve together, not to dominate the opponent.

Getting Started with Sparring:

• **Warm-Up:** Prior to sparring, practitioners should engage in a thorough warm-up to prepare their bodies and prevent injuries.

• **Drills:** Practicing specific drills can help students refine techniques and build confidence before engaging in sparring.

• **Start Slow:** Beginners should start with controlled sparring, gradually increasing intensity as they become more comfortable and proficient.

• **Feedback:** After sparring sessions, practitioners should seek feedback from instructors and partners to identify areas for improvement and adjust their strategies.

Sparring is an essential component of training in Shaolin Kempo Karate, providing practitioners with valuable opportunities to apply techniques, enhance skills, and develop strategic thinking. Through regular sparring practice, students build confidence, improve physical conditioning, and prepare for real-life self-defense situations and competition. Emphasizing safety, respect, and sportsmanship ensures that sparring remains a constructive and enjoyable aspect of martial arts training.

Sparring Drills

Sparring drills are essential for developing the skills, techniques, and mental strategies necessary for effective sparring in Shaolin Kempo Karate. These drills help practitioners refine their movements, improve their timing and distance control, and build confidence in a controlled setting. Below are some effective sparring drills suitable for various skill levels:

1. Shadow Sparring:

• **Objective:** To practice techniques and combinations without a partner.

How to Perform:

• Visualize an opponent and practice various strikes, blocks, and footwork.

• Focus on fluidity and form while incorporating movement and combinations.

• Work on different angles, speeds, and rhythms.

2. Partner Drills:

• **Objective:** To practice specific techniques with a partner in a controlled manner.

How to Perform:

• **Basic Combinations:** One partner throws a set combination (e.g., jab-cross-hook), while the other defends and counters.

• **Block and Counter:** One partner attacks with a specific strike (e.g., front kick), while the other practices blocking and immediately countering with a designated technique.

• **Predetermined Sparring:** Partners agree on a set of techniques to use (e.g., only punches or kicks) to focus on applying specific skills.

3. Distance Management Drills:

• **Objective:** To enhance distance control and movement.

How to Perform:

• One partner attacks while the other practices stepping back or to the side to evade strikes.

• Focus on maintaining proper distance to launch counterattacks effectively.

• Switch roles to allow both partners to practice offensive and defensive movements.

4. Footwork Drills:

- **Objective:** To improve agility and movement during sparring.

How to Perform:

• Set up cones or markers in a square or circle. Practitioners move in and out, practicing footwork while maintaining guard.

• Incorporate various footwork patterns (e.g., shuffling, circling, advancing, retreating) to simulate real sparring scenarios.

• Add a partner who can attack or feint to challenge the moving partner to respond appropriately.

5. Controlled Sparring:

• **Objective:** To practice sparring in a controlled environment with specific rules.

How to Perform:

• Set a timer (e.g., 1-2 minutes) and engage in light sparring with an emphasis on technique rather than power.

• Focus on using specific techniques or combinations during the sparring session (e.g., only upper body strikes).

• Instructors can provide feedback after each round to enhance learning.

6. Reaction Drills:

• **Objective:** To improve reflexes and quick responses.

How to Perform:

• One partner randomly throws strikes (e.g., punches or kicks) at a controlled speed while the other practices reacting with appropriate blocks or evasive movements.

• Focus on maintaining composure and timing responses accurately.

• Switch roles after a set time or number of attacks.

7. Conditioning Sparring:

• **Objective:** To enhance physical conditioning while practicing sparring techniques.

How to Perform:

- Engage in continuous sparring for a set time (e.g., 3-5 minutes) with light to moderate contact.

• Partners can take turns attacking and defending, encouraging the use of movement and combinations throughout.

• Emphasize maintaining stamina and technique under fatigue.

8. Counter-Sparring Drills:

• **Objective:** To practice counterattacks after successfully defending against an opponent's strike.

How to Perform:

• One partner attacks with a specific strike (e.g., jab), and the other practices defending (e.g., blocking) and immediately countering.

• Switch roles to allow both partners to experience attacking and defending.

• Focus on timing, precision, and following up after the defense.

Sparring drills are crucial for developing the skills and confidence needed for effective sparring in Shaolin Kempo Karate. By incorporating various drills into training, practitioners can refine their techniques, enhance their physical conditioning, and prepare for real sparring scenarios. Regular practice of these drills will improve overall performance and readiness for competitive and self-defense situations.

Sparring Strategies And Techniques

Sparring strategies and techniques are essential for effective performance in sparring sessions, competitions, or self-defense situations in Shaolin Kempo Karate. By understanding how to apply various techniques and adapt to different scenarios, practitioners can enhance their effectiveness and develop a strategic mindset. Here's an overview of key sparring strategies and techniques:

Sparring Strategies

Understanding Distance and Timing:

- **Maintain Proper Distance:** Learn to judge the distance between you and your opponent to effectively launch attacks or evade strikes. Use footwork to create the optimal distance for your techniques.

• **Timing is Key:** Observe your opponent's movements to anticipate their attacks. Timing your strikes just as they commit to their attack can increase your chances of landing a successful counter.

Offensive and Defensive Balance:

• **Mixing Offense and Defense:** Striking while simultaneously defending creates an effective strategy. Use blocks to absorb attacks while positioning yourself for counterattacks.

• **Use Feints:** Feinting can mislead your opponent into thinking you are attacking one area, allowing you to strike in a different direction when they commit to a defense.

Adapting to Your Opponent:

• **Read Their Style:** Pay attention to your opponent's techniques and tendencies.

Adapt your strategy based on their strengths and weaknesses, such as focusing on defending against their preferred strikes.

• **Stay Unpredictable:** Vary your attacks and movements to keep your opponent guessing. Switching between high and low attacks, or using different techniques, can create openings for successful strikes.

Utilizing Combinations:

• **Develop Effective Combinations:** Practice and implement combinations of strikes and techniques. For example, follow a punch with a kick or a knee strike to increase your chances of success.

• **Quick Successions:** Use rapid combinations to overwhelm your opponent and break through their defenses.

Positioning and Angles:

• **Use Angles to Your Advantage:** Move at angles to create openings and avoid direct confrontations. This can make it difficult for your opponent to land effective strikes while giving you better positioning for your attacks.

• **Control the Center Line:** Try to maintain control of the center line, where your opponent's attacks are most direct. This positioning can provide a tactical advantage in terms of control and defensive opportunities.

Techniques for Sparring

Basic Strikes:

• **Jab (Tsuki):** A quick and direct punch used to gauge distance or disrupt your opponent's rhythm.

- **Cross (Chudan Tsuki):** A powerful straight punch that follows the jab, targeting the opponent's head or torso.

- **Hook (Ura Tsuki):** A side punch that targets the head or body, effective for breaking through defenses.

Kicking Techniques:

- **Front Kick (Mae Geri):** A direct kick aimed at the opponent's body or head, effective for creating distance.

- **Roundhouse Kick (Mawashi Geri):** A versatile kick targeting the head or ribs, effective for both offense and defense.

- **Side Kick (Yoko Geri):** A powerful kick used to push back or disrupt an opponent's balance.

Defensive Techniques:

• **Blocking (Uke):** Use various blocking techniques (e.g., high block, low block) to defend against strikes.

• **Parrying:** Redirect an incoming attack with a quick motion, setting yourself up for a counter.

• **Evasion:** Utilize footwork to step back, sidestep, or angle away from attacks to avoid strikes entirely.

Counterattacks:

• **Immediate Counter:** As your opponent strikes, use their momentum against them by blocking or evading and immediately countering.

• **Delayed Counter:** Allow your opponent to commit to their attack before launching a counter, creating an opportunity as they expose themselves.

Clinch and Grappling Techniques:

• **Clinch Fighting:** Get close to your opponent to neutralize their striking capabilities and create opportunities for knee strikes or throws.

• **Joint Locks and Takedowns:** Use basic grappling techniques to off-balance your opponent and control the situation when in close range.

Incorporating effective sparring strategies and techniques in Shaolin Kempo Karate enhances a practitioner's ability to perform well in sparring sessions and self-defense situations.

By understanding distance, timing, and adapting to opponents, as well as utilizing a diverse range of strikes and defensive techniques, practitioners can become more confident and proficient in their martial arts practice. Regular sparring practice, combined with the application of these strategies and techniques, will lead to improved performance and readiness for various combat scenarios.

Safety And Etiquette In Sparring

Safety and etiquette in sparring are crucial for creating a positive and constructive training environment in Shaolin Kempo Karate. Adhering to safety protocols and respectful behavior not only minimizes the risk of injury but also fosters a sense of camaraderie and mutual respect among practitioners. Here are key aspects of safety and etiquette to consider during sparring sessions:

Safety in Sparring

Protective Gear

Always wear appropriate protective equipment, such as:

- **Headgear:** To protect the head and face from strikes.

- **Mouthguard:** To prevent dental injuries.

- **Gloves:** To protect the hands and reduce the impact on your partner.

- **Shin Guards:** To protect the shins during kicks.

- **Chest Protectors:** To shield the torso from powerful strikes.

Ensure that all protective gear is properly fitted and in good condition.

Controlled Environment:

• Sparring should be conducted in a safe, supervised setting. Instructors should oversee the sessions to ensure adherence to safety guidelines.

• Use a suitable training surface, such as a padded mat, to minimize the risk of injury from falls.

Understanding Intensity Levels:

• Communicate with your sparring partner to agree on the intensity level of the sparring session (e.g., light, medium, or full contact).

• Adjust your techniques based on the agreed intensity to prevent injuries. For example, use lighter strikes during controlled sparring.

Focus on Technique:

• Emphasize technique and control over power. Practicing techniques with control reduces the risk of accidents and injuries.

• Avoid reckless behavior, such as swinging wildly or throwing hard punches without regard for your partner's safety.

Stay Aware of Your Surroundings

• Maintain awareness of your surroundings, including the location of other practitioners, equipment, and barriers.

• If sparring near other pairs, ensure enough space to avoid collisions.

Warm-Up and Cool Down:

• Engage in a proper warm-up before sparring to prepare the body and reduce the risk of injury.

• Cool down after sparring to aid recovery and prevent muscle soreness.

Etiquette in Sparring

Respect Your Partner:

• Treat your sparring partner with respect, regardless of their skill level. Sparring is a cooperative practice, and mutual respect enhances the learning experience.

• Avoid taunting or belittling your partner, as this can create a hostile atmosphere.

Communicate Openly:

• Before sparring, discuss any concerns, preferences, or limitations with your partner. This ensures both parties are comfortable and on the same page.

• After the sparring session, provide constructive feedback and discuss areas for improvement.

Practice Sportsmanship:

• Display good sportsmanship by congratulating your partner after a sparring session, regardless of the outcome.

• Avoid arguing or showing frustration after being scored upon or bested in sparring.

Be a Good Listener:

• Listen to your instructor and follow their guidance during sparring sessions. They provide valuable insights and ensure the safety and effectiveness of the training.

• Be open to feedback from instructors and partners to improve your skills and understanding.

Stay Humble:

• Maintain humility in victory and graciousness in defeat. Every sparring session is an opportunity to learn, regardless of the outcome.

• Focus on personal improvement rather than solely on winning.

Follow the Rules:

• Adhere to the established rules and guidelines for sparring within your dojo or training facility. These rules are designed to ensure a safe and productive environment for all practitioners.

Safety and etiquette are essential components of sparring in Shaolin Kempo Karate. By prioritizing protective measures, maintaining a respectful attitude towards partners, and fostering a supportive training atmosphere, practitioners can enhance their sparring experience. Adhering to these principles will not only minimize the risk of injury but also promote personal growth, camaraderie, and a positive martial arts community.

CHAPTER 5: SELF-DEFENSE APPLICATIONS

Principles Of Self-Defense

The principles of self-defense are fundamental guidelines that help practitioners effectively protect themselves in threatening situations. In Shaolin Kempo Karate, these principles emphasize not just physical techniques but also mental preparedness and situational awareness. Here are key principles of self-defense:

1. Awareness and Prevention:

• **Stay Alert:** Always be aware of your surroundings and the people around you. This heightened awareness can help you identify potential threats before they escalate.

• **Trust Your Instincts:** If something feels off or you sense danger, trust your instincts and take proactive measures to avoid confrontation.

• **Avoidance:** Whenever possible, avoid conflict. De-escalate situations through verbal communication, and retreat from potentially dangerous environments.

2. Use of the Environment:

• **Utilize Your Surroundings:** Be aware of objects in your environment that can be used for defense or to create distance (e.g., doors, furniture, and barriers).

• **Escape Routes:** Always have an escape route in mind. If a confrontation occurs, seek an opportunity to safely exit the situation.

3. De-escalation Techniques:

• **Verbal Communication:** Use calm and assertive language to defuse a situation. Engage in dialogue to redirect aggressive behavior and create a peaceful resolution.

• **Non-threatening Body Language:** Maintain an open and relaxed posture to reduce tension and avoid provoking aggression.

4. Effective Techniques:

• **Target Vulnerable Areas:** Focus on vulnerable areas of the attacker's body (e.g., eyes, throat, groin) when countering an attack. Striking these areas can create opportunities to escape.

• **Leverage and Control:** Use techniques that allow you to leverage your opponent's force against them. Joint locks and throws can neutralize an attacker effectively without requiring excessive strength.

5. Control and Restraint:

• **Proportional Response:** Your response should be proportional to the threat level. Use minimal force necessary to protect yourself and create an opportunity to escape.

• **Avoid Excessive Force:** Once you have neutralized the threat and have an opportunity to escape, refrain from pursuing further aggression.

6. Mental Preparedness:

• **Stay Calm:** Maintaining composure under pressure is vital. Practice breathing techniques and visualization to help manage stress during confrontations.

• **Mindset:** Develop a confident and assertive mindset. Believing in your ability to defend yourself can enhance your effectiveness in a threatening situation.

7. Training and Practice:

• **Regular Training:** Consistently practice self-defense techniques through drills and sparring to build muscle memory and confidence.

• **Scenario Training:** Engage in realistic self-defense scenarios to improve your response to various situations and increase your adaptability.

8. Legal Considerations:

• **Know Your Rights:** Familiarize yourself with local laws regarding self-defense. Understand the legal implications of using force in self-defense situations.

- **Document Incidents:** In the event of a confrontation, document what happened as soon as possible, noting details that may be relevant for legal purposes.

The principles of self-defense in Shaolin Kempo Karate encompass awareness, avoidance, effective techniques, and mental preparedness. By understanding and applying these principles, practitioners can enhance their ability to protect themselves while fostering a mindset focused on de-escalation and safety. Regular training, awareness, and a calm approach are key elements in developing effective self-defense skills.

Techniques For Common Attacks

In Shaolin Kempo Karate, knowing how to respond effectively to common attacks is essential for self-defense. Practitioners learn techniques to counter various types of attacks, focusing on using leverage, speed, and precision. Here are some techniques for responding to common attacks:

1. Defense Against Punches

Straight Punch (Jab/Cross)

Technique:

• **Block and Counter:** Use a high block (jodan uke) with your lead hand to deflect the punch while simultaneously stepping offline to create an angle. Follow up with a counter punch to the opponent's face or body.

• **Slip and Counter:** Move your head slightly to the side to evade the punch while launching a quick counterattack to the body or head.

Hook Punch

Technique:

• **Duck and Counter:** Bend your knees and lower your body to slip under the hook while delivering a quick uppercut or straight punch to the opponent's chin.

• **Parry and Counter:** Use your rear hand to parry the punch away from your face while stepping offline, then immediately counter with a straight punch or kick.

2. Defense Against Kicks

Front Kick

Technique:

• **Catch and Counter:** If the kick is directed toward your body, catch the opponent's kicking leg with both hands and pull them off balance, then counter with a strike or sweep.

• **Side Step and Counter:** Step offline to evade the kick while delivering a counter punch to the opponent's head or body.

Roundhouse Kick

Technique:

• **Block and Counter:** Use a low block (gedan uke) with your lead arm to deflect the kick. As you block, pivot on your lead foot to create distance and follow up with a counter kick or punch.

• **Evade and Counter:** Lean back or side step to evade the kick, creating an opportunity to counter with a front kick or a side kick to the opponent's body.

3. Defense Against Grabs

Wrist Grab

Technique:

• **Twist and Escape:** Rotate your wrist toward the opponent's thumb (the weakest part of their grip) while stepping back to create distance. This can loosen their grip and allow you to escape.

• **Counter with a Strike:** As you twist your wrist free, deliver an immediate strike (e.g., elbow or knee) to the opponent's face or torso.

Clothes Grab

Technique:

• **Pull and Strike:** Use the opponent's grip to your advantage by pulling them forward while delivering a strike (e.g., knee or punch) to their face or body.

• **Joint Lock:** Apply a wrist lock or shoulder lock to control the opponent's arm, neutralizing their ability to attack further.

4. Defense Against Chokes

Front Choke (Two Hands)

Technique:

• **Tuck and Turn:** Tuck your chin down to protect your throat, then step to the side while driving your shoulder into the attacker's chest. Use your hands to break the grip while following up with a knee strike to the groin or a punch.

• **Escape and Counter:** Use your arms to create space, then turn and deliver a strike (e.g., elbow or knee) to escape the choke.

Rear Choke (Two Hands)

Technique:

• **Drop and Roll:** If caught from behind, drop your weight and roll to one side while pushing against their arm, breaking the choke. Follow up with a strike to the attacker's head or ribs as you escape.

• **Hand Defense:** Bring your hands up to protect your neck and create space by pushing against their arms. Use your body to turn into them, delivering an elbow strike or knee to the groin.

5. Defense Against Takedowns

Single Leg Takedown

Technique:

• **Sprawl:** When your opponent attempts to grab your leg, sprawl your body back and down to prevent them from completing the takedown. Use your hands to push down on their shoulders or head while establishing a dominant position.

• **Counter with a Strike:** As they attempt the takedown, maintain your balance and deliver a knee strike to the opponent's head or body.

Double Leg Takedown

Technique:

• **Wide Stance and Defense:** Widen your stance to lower your center of gravity and use your arms to push down on their shoulders. Keep your hips back to maintain balance.

• **Underhook and Counter:** As they attempt the takedown, use an underhook on one side to lift and control their body, creating space for a knee strike or escape.

Effective self-defense techniques for common attacks in Shaolin Kempo Karate focus on using leverage, speed, and strategic thinking. By mastering these techniques, practitioners can enhance their ability to respond to various threats and protect themselves in real-life situations. Regular practice and scenario training will help build confidence and improve response times in the face of an attack.

CHAPTER 6: ADVANCED TECHNIQUES
Advanced Blocks And Strikes

In Shaolin Kempo Karate, advanced blocks and strikes are essential components for developing effective self-defense techniques and improving overall martial arts proficiency. These techniques require proper execution, timing, and precision. Here's an overview of some advanced blocks and strikes:

Advanced Blocks

X-Block (Cross Block):

• **Description:** An advanced block used to defend against simultaneous attacks from multiple angles.

Execution:

• Cross your forearms in front of your body, creating an "X" shape to block incoming strikes from both sides.

• Keep your elbows close to your body and your hands high to protect your head and upper body.

Inside Block (Uchi Uke);

• **Description:** An effective block for deflecting attacks coming from the outside.

Execution:

• Raise your lead arm to deflect an incoming strike inward while pivoting on your back foot to create an angle.

• Use your other hand to prepare for a counterattack.

Outside Block (Soto Uke):

• **Description:** A versatile block that deflects incoming strikes from the inside.

Execution:

• Extend your arm outward to deflect an incoming punch or kick, rotating your body for additional power.

• Maintain a strong stance to absorb the impact while preparing to counter.

Palm Block (Tate Uke):

• **Description:** A defensive technique used to block high attacks.

Execution:

• Raise your palm vertically to deflect strikes aimed at your head, ensuring your elbow is slightly bent.

- Follow through by transitioning into a counterattack with a strike.

Knee Block (Hiza Uke):

- **Description:** A block used to defend against low attacks or kicks to the lower body.

Execution:

- Raise your knee to intercept the attack while shifting your weight back to maintain balance.

- Transition into a counter technique, such as a kick or punch, immediately after blocking.

Advanced Strikes

Backfist Strike (Uraken):

• **Description:** A quick, powerful strike delivered using the back of the fist.

Execution:

• Rotate your body and pivot on your lead foot as you extend your arm, striking with the back of your fist to the opponent's face or head.

• Use a snapping motion to maximize impact.

Elbow Strike (Hiji Ate):

• **Description:** A close-range strike that utilizes the elbow to deliver powerful impacts.

Execution:

• Pivot your body and bring your elbow sharply down or across to strike the opponent's face, ribs, or temple.

• Keep your guard up to protect yourself while executing the strike.

Knee Strike (Hiza Geri):

• **Description:** An effective technique for striking opponents at close range.

Execution:

• Lift your knee sharply to target the opponent's midsection or chin, driving your weight forward for additional power.

• Follow up with other techniques as needed, such as punches or kicks.

Hammer Fist Strike (Tate Uraken):

• **Description:** A downward strike delivered with the bottom of the fist, effective against a variety of targets.

Execution:

• Raise your fist above your shoulder and bring it down forcefully to strike the opponent's head, collarbone, or other vulnerable areas.

• Rotate your hips and shoulders to generate power.

Side Kick (Yoko Geri)

• **Description:** A powerful kick that targets the opponent's torso or head from the side.

Execution:

• Pivot on your supporting foot, lifting your knee high and extending your leg sideways.

• Strike with the heel or side of the foot, ensuring your body is balanced and your posture is correct to absorb any counterattacks.

Roundhouse Kick (Mawashi Geri):

• **Description:** A versatile kick targeting the opponent's head or body with a circular motion.

Execution:

• Lift your knee and pivot on your support foot, swinging your leg in a circular motion to strike with the instep or shin.

• Maintain balance throughout the kick, using your arms for support and balance.

Advanced blocks and strikes in Shaolin Kempo Karate play a crucial role in enhancing self-defense capabilities and overall martial arts proficiency. Practitioners should focus on proper technique, timing, and integration of these advanced techniques into their sparring and self-defense practice. Regular training and application of these techniques will lead to improved skill and effectiveness in various combat scenarios.

Joint Locks And Manipulations

Joint locks and manipulations are essential techniques in Shaolin Kempo Karate and other martial arts. These techniques allow practitioners to control or incapacitate an opponent by targeting specific joints, leveraging their anatomy against them. Here's an overview of some common joint locks and manipulations, along with their applications:

Principles of Joint Locks

• **Leverage and Control**: Joint locks rely on using leverage to control an opponent's movements. By applying pressure to specific joints, you can limit their ability to resist or escape.

• **Pain Compliance**: Many joint locks create discomfort or pain in the opponent, encouraging them to comply with your commands or release their hold.

• **Positioning**: Effective joint locks often require proper positioning and body alignment. Use your body weight and hip movement to maximize the effectiveness of the lock.

• **Safety**: Always practice joint locks with caution to prevent injury to your training partners. Start slowly and gradually increase intensity as proficiency improves.

Common Joint Locks and Manipulations

Wrist Lock (Kote Gaeshi):

• **Description:** A technique used to control the opponent's wrist by applying pressure to the joint.

Execution:

• Grasp the opponent's wrist with one hand, rotating it inward while pushing their elbow down.

• Maintain control of their arm, applying pressure to the wrist joint to immobilize them.

Elbow Lock (Hiji Gamae):

• **Description:** A technique targeting the elbow joint, often used to control or take down an opponent.

Execution:

• Grab the opponent's arm and bend it at the elbow, using your other hand to push down on their forearm.

• Rotate their wrist while keeping the elbow bent to increase pressure on the joint.

Shoulder Lock (Ushiro Gamae):

• **Description:** A control technique targeting the shoulder joint, effective for immobilizing an opponent.

Execution:

• Grasp the opponent's arm and pull it behind their back while pressing downward on their shoulder.

• Keep your body close to theirs for leverage, maintaining pressure to restrict their movement.

Finger Lock (Yubi Gamae):

• **Description:** A manipulation that targets the fingers to control an opponent's hand.

Execution:

• Grasp one or more of the opponent's fingers and bend them backward while controlling their wrist.

• Use your body position to maintain balance and leverage while applying pressure.

Hip Throw (O Goshi):

• **Description:** While primarily a throw, the hip throw can incorporate joint locking principles.

Execution:

• Secure a grip on the opponent's waist and turn your hips to lift them over your hip while controlling their arm.

• This technique can be enhanced with an elbow lock as they fall.

Knee Lock (Hiza Gamae):

• **Description:** A technique that targets the knee joint, often used in self-defense scenarios.

Execution:

• Position yourself to apply pressure to the opponent's knee while controlling their upper body.

• Use your body weight to push down on the knee, creating discomfort or immobilization.

Ankle Lock (Ashi Uke):

• **Description:** A technique targeting the ankle joint, effective for taking down an opponent.

Execution:

• Control the opponent's foot and ankle by lifting and twisting it outward, applying pressure to the joint.

• This can be combined with a takedown for greater effectiveness.

Applications of Joint Locks:

• **Self-Defense**: Joint locks can effectively incapacitate an aggressor or create opportunities to escape dangerous situations.

• **Controlling an Opponent**: In a sparring or competition context, joint locks can be used to control the opponent's movements and limit their ability to strike or escape.

• **Submissions in Grappling**: Many joint locks are commonly used in grappling sports (e.g., Brazilian Jiu-Jitsu, Judo) as submission techniques to force opponents to submit.

Physical Restraint: Joint locks can be used by law enforcement or security personnel to safely restrain individuals without causing serious injury.

Joint locks and manipulations are vital components of Shaolin Kempo Karate, offering practitioners a range of techniques for controlling and incapacitating opponents. By mastering these techniques, practitioners can enhance their self-defense skills and overall effectiveness in martial arts. Regular practice, attention to detail, and a focus on safety are crucial for developing proficiency in joint locks and manipulations.

Throws And Takedowns

Throws and takedowns are integral parts of Shaolin Kempo Karate and many other martial arts. They allow practitioners to leverage balance, body weight, and technique to control or incapacitate an opponent. Understanding the principles behind these techniques can enhance your overall effectiveness in self-defense and sparring. Here's an overview of some common throws and takedowns, including their execution and applications:

Principles of Throws and Takedowns:

• **Leverage and Balance:** Throws and takedowns rely on using your opponent's weight and balance against them. By shifting their center of gravity, you can execute a successful technique.

• **Body Positioning:** Proper body positioning is crucial. You should always be aware of your stance and how to position your body relative to your opponent.

• **Timing and Coordination**: Executing throws and takedowns effectively requires precise timing and coordination. Recognize your opponent's movements and respond accordingly.

• **Control and Safety**: Always practice throws and takedowns safely. Use controlled movements to avoid injury to yourself and your training partner.

Common Throws

Hip Throw (O Goshi):

• **Description:** A fundamental throw that uses the hips to lift and throw the opponent.

Execution:

• Step in close to your opponent and secure a grip around their waist.

• Pivot on your lead foot, turning your back to them while lowering your hips.

• Lift with your hips and throw them over your shoulder, using their momentum to assist in the throw.

Shoulder Throw (Seoi Nage):

• **Description:** A powerful throw that utilizes the shoulder to project the opponent.

Execution:

• Secure a grip on the opponent's arm and step to the side.

• Lower your body, positioning your shoulder under their center of gravity.

• Pull them over your shoulder while rotating your body, allowing gravity to assist the throw.

Throwing Knee (Knee Throw):

• **Description:** A technique that combines a knee strike with a throw.

Execution:

• As you strike your opponent with a knee to their midsection, use your other hand to control their upper body.

• Lean back slightly and pivot, throwing them off balance and using their momentum to complete the throw.

Foot Sweep (Ashi Barai):

• **Description:** A low throw that targets the opponent's feet to trip them.

Execution:

• Step close to your opponent and pivot on your lead foot.

• Use your rear foot to sweep their foot or leg while maintaining upper body control.

• Follow through to ensure they lose balance and fall.

Body Drop (Tai Otoshi):

• **Description:** A technique that uses body weight to drop the opponent to the ground.

Execution:

• Position your body in front of the opponent, then shift your weight onto one leg.

• Use your other leg to hook behind their leg while pulling them down and forward with your arms.

• Ensure that you control their fall to prevent injury.

Common Takedowns

Single-Leg Takedown:

• **Description:** A technique that targets one of the opponent's legs to bring them down.

Execution:

• Close the distance and lower your body to grab one of their legs, ideally around the knee or ankle.

• Drive forward while lifting the leg, causing the opponent to lose balance and fall.

• Use your body to create a barrier to prevent them from escaping.

Double-Leg Takedown

• **Description:** A more aggressive takedown that targets both legs.

Execution:

• Lower your body and position yourself between the opponent's legs.

• Wrap your arms around their thighs and lift while driving forward.

• Use your momentum to take them down to the ground.

Ouchi Gari (Major Inner Reap):

• **Description:** A takedown that targets the inside of the opponent's legs.

Execution:

- Step off to the side and sweep one of your opponent's legs with your leg while pushing them backward.

- Use your hands to control their upper body for balance and leverage.

- Ensure the sweeping motion is quick and fluid.

Kouchi Gari (Minor Inner Reap):

- **Description:** Similar to Ouchi Gari but targets the opponent's other leg with a smaller sweeping motion.

Execution:

- Position yourself similarly to the Ouchi Gari, but target the opposite leg.

- Sweep the leg with your foot while pushing the upper body back for a clean takedown.

<u>**Applications of Throws and Takedowns:**</u>

• **Self-Defense**: Throws and takedowns can effectively neutralize an attacker by taking them off their feet, creating an opportunity for escape.

• **Competition and Sparring**: In a competitive context, throws and takedowns are used to score points and control opponents, demonstrating technical proficiency and strategy.

• **Grappling and Ground Fighting**: Throws and takedowns transition smoothly into grappling scenarios, allowing practitioners to maintain control on the ground.

• **Control and Restraint**: Law enforcement or security personnel can use these techniques to safely restrain individuals without causing injury.

Throws and takedowns are powerful techniques in Shaolin Kempo Karate that rely on leverage, timing, and body positioning. By mastering these techniques, practitioners can enhance their self-defense capabilities and overall martial arts proficiency. Regular practice, attention to detail, and a focus on safety will contribute to successful execution in various combat scenarios.

Pressure Points

Pressure points are specific areas of the body that are sensitive to touch or pressure and can be used effectively in self-defense and martial arts, including Shaolin Kempo Karate. Knowledge of these points allows practitioners to incapacitate an opponent, manage pain, or control movement. Here's an overview of pressure points, their locations, and applications:

<u>Understanding Pressure Points</u>

• **Anatomy and Physiology:** Pressure points correspond to areas where nerves, blood vessels, and tissues are densely packed. Stimulating these points can disrupt the body's normal function and induce pain or disorientation.

• **Pain Compliance**: Targeting pressure points can lead to pain compliance, where an opponent is compelled to submit or change their behavior due to discomfort.

• **Control and Manipulation**: Pressure points can be used to control an opponent's movements, making them useful in self-defense scenarios and grappling.

• **Focus and Precision**: Effective use of pressure points requires precision and understanding of body mechanics. Strikes should be quick and focused for maximum effect.

Common Pressure Points and Their Applications

Temple (Shin Ten):

• **Location:** Located on the side of the head, just above the ear.

• **Application:** A strong strike or pressure applied to this area can cause dizziness, confusion, or unconsciousness.

Jaw (Mandibular Angle):

• **Location:** The area where the jaw meets the skull, just below the ear.

• **Application:** Striking or applying pressure here can cause disorientation and pain, making it an effective target for a quick finish.

Throat (Carotid Artery):

• **Location:** The center of the neck, just below the Adam's apple.

• **Application:** Striking the throat can disrupt breathing and create panic in the opponent. However, it should be used with caution due to the potential for serious injury.

Solar Plexus:

• **Location:** Located in the center of the abdomen, just below the ribcage.

• **Application:** A strike to this area can cause severe pain and temporarily incapacitate the opponent by disrupting their breath.

Ribs (Floating Ribs):

• **Location:** The lower ribs that do not connect to the sternum.

• **Application:** Striking or applying pressure to these ribs can cause significant pain and difficulty in breathing, making them effective targets in self-defense.

Elbow (Ulnar Nerve):

• **Location:** The nerve located on the inside of the elbow.

• **Application:** A sharp strike or pressure can cause intense pain and temporary loss of control over the arm.

Wrist (Carpal Tunnel):

• **Location:** The area where the wrist bones are located, especially on the underside.

• **Application:** Applying pressure here can immobilize the hand or cause pain, making it a strategic target in joint locks or grappling.

Knee (Patellar Tendon):

• **Location:** Just below the kneecap.

• **Application:** Striking this area can destabilize the opponent and cause pain, making it effective for takedowns or creating an opportunity to escape.

Inner Thigh (Femoral Nerve)

• **Location:** The inner thigh, where the femoral nerve runs.

• **Application:** A strike or pressure here can cause significant pain and disrupt balance, making it a useful target in close combat.

Applications of Pressure Points in Self-Defense

• **Incapacitation**: Using pressure points effectively can incapacitate an opponent, providing an opportunity to escape or seek help.

• **Control and Restraint**: Pressure points can be used to control an opponent's movements, allowing for easier restraint or management of the situation.

• **Pain Compliance**: Striking pressure points can induce pain, leading to compliance from the opponent without the need for excessive force.

• **Disruption of Movement**: Targeting specific pressure points can disrupt the opponent's ability to move effectively, providing an advantage in a confrontation.

Understanding pressure points in Shaolin Kempo Karate enhances a practitioner's self-defense toolkit, providing effective techniques for incapacitating or controlling an opponent.

Training should focus on precision, control, and safety to ensure responsible application of these techniques in practice and real-life situations. Regular practice and application will lead to improved skill and confidence in using pressure points effectively.

CHAPTER 7: WEAPONS TRAINING
History And Philosophy Of Weapons In Shaolin Kempo Karate

The history and philosophy of weapons in Shaolin Kempo Karate reflect a rich cultural heritage rooted in traditional martial arts. Understanding this history enhances practitioners' appreciation of the techniques and their applications. Here's an overview of the historical context, evolution, and philosophical principles behind weapons training in Shaolin Kempo Karate.

Monks at the temple developed various combat techniques, integrating philosophy and spirituality into their practice, which included unarmed combat as well as weapons training.

Shaolin Kempo Karate draws heavily from traditional Chinese martial arts, which have a long history of weaponry. Weapons such as the staff (gun), sword (jian), and spear (qiang) were incorporated into martial training to enhance combat effectiveness and discipline.

The blending of these styles into the development of Kempo reflects the historical significance of weapon training in martial arts culture.

Introduction of Japanese Influence:

Kempo, meaning "fist law," has roots in both Chinese martial arts and Japanese systems. When Kempo spread to Japan, various weapons techniques were adopted, contributing to the evolution of modern Kempo styles, including Shaolin Kempo Karate.

The Japanese influence brought techniques and philosophies from various schools of martial arts, further enriching the weapon training curriculum.

Over time, Shaolin Kempo Karate integrated various weapons into its training, focusing on both traditional and modern applications. Common weapons taught in Shaolin Kempo include the staff (bo), nunchaku, sai, and katana, each offering unique techniques and strategies for combat.

Philosophical Principles:

• **Harmony and Balance**: The philosophy behind weapons training in Shaolin Kempo Karate emphasizes harmony between the practitioner and the weapon. Understanding the weapon's dynamics and integrating it into one's body movements are crucial for effective use. Practitioners learn to maintain balance and control while wielding a weapon, reflecting the importance of harmony in both martial arts and life.

• **Discipline and Respect**: Weapons training requires a high level of discipline and respect, both for the weapon and for oneself. Practitioners are taught to handle weapons with care and to understand the responsibilities that come with wielding them. This discipline extends to respect for opponents and the martial arts community, emphasizing humility and honor.

• **Mindfulness and Focus**: The practice of using weapons demands concentration and mindfulness. Practitioners must be fully present in their movements, fostering a deeper connection between mind and body. This focus is not only essential for effective training but also promotes mental clarity and emotional stability.

- **Self-Defense and Responsibility**: Weapons training in Shaolin Kempo Karate is rooted in self-defense. Practitioners are taught to use weapons responsibly, emphasizing that they should only be employed in legitimate self-defense situations. The philosophy encourages practitioners to seek peaceful resolutions before resorting to violence, reinforcing the martial arts' core values of non-aggression.

- **Integration of Techniques**: Weapons training is integrated with empty-hand techniques, encouraging practitioners to adapt their skills depending on the situation. This holistic approach teaches that a weapon can be an extension of the body, promoting fluidity in movement and adaptability in combat scenarios.

The history and philosophy of weapons in Shaolin Kempo Karate are deeply intertwined with its origins and development as a martial art. By understanding this context, practitioners can appreciate the significance of weapons training as a means of personal growth, discipline, and self-defense.

Emphasizing harmony, respect, mindfulness, and responsibility, the philosophy of weapons training enriches the overall martial arts experience and fosters a deeper connection between practitioners and their art. Regular training and study of these principles will enhance skill, understanding, and appreciation for the rich heritage of Shaolin Kempo Karate.

Basic Weapons

Basic weapons training is an integral part of Shaolin Kempo Karate, allowing practitioners to develop their skills and understanding of martial arts. Each weapon offers unique techniques and applications, enhancing both self-defense capabilities and the overall martial arts experience. Here's an overview of some common basic weapons used in Shaolin Kempo Karate, including their descriptions, techniques, and applications:

1. Bo Staff:

• **Description:** The bo staff is a long, wooden staff typically measuring around 6 feet in length. It is a versatile weapon used for striking, blocking, and thrusting.

Techniques:

• **Strikes:** Various strikes can be delivered from different angles, including downward, upward, and horizontal strikes.

• **Blocks:** The staff can be used to deflect incoming attacks, providing a defensive advantage.

• **Thrusts:** Forward thrusts target specific points, effectively creating distance from an opponent.

• **Applications:** The bo staff is excellent for developing coordination, timing, and distance management. It is often used in forms, sparring, and self-defense scenarios.

2. Nunchaku:

• **Description:** Nunchaku consists of two sticks connected by a short chain or rope.

This weapon requires dexterity and practice to master its techniques.

Techniques:

• **Striking:** The ends of the nunchaku can deliver powerful strikes to various target areas, including the head, limbs, and torso.

• **Spinning:** Practitioners can spin the nunchaku around their hands and body for both defensive and offensive maneuvers.

• **Locking:** The nunchaku can be used to entrap an opponent's limbs, controlling their movements.

• **Applications:** Nunchaku training enhances hand-eye coordination, timing, and fluidity of movement. It is often practiced in forms and demonstrations.

3. Sai

• **Description:** The sai is a traditional Okinawan weapon resembling a three-pronged dagger, typically made of metal. It is used for thrusting, striking, and trapping.

Techniques:

• **Thrusts:** Direct thrusts target vital points, creating effective offensive maneuvers.

• **Blocks:** The sai can be used to block or redirect incoming attacks, providing a defensive advantage.

• **Trapping:** The middle prong can trap an opponent's weapon or limb, allowing for control and follow-up techniques.

• **Applications:** Sai training develops precision, agility, and understanding of angles. Practitioners often incorporate sai into forms and self-defense techniques.

4. Katana

• **Description:** The katana is a traditional Japanese sword known for its curved, single-edged blade. It is revered for its cutting ability and precision.

Techniques:

• **Cuts:** Various cutting techniques, including downward, diagonal, and upward cuts, are essential for effective use.

• **Thrusts:** The katana can also be used for thrusting attacks, targeting vital points.

• **Defensive Techniques:** Practitioners learn to use the blade defensively to parry and block incoming attacks.

• **Applications:** Katana training emphasizes precision, discipline, and control. It is often practiced in kata (forms) and sparring scenarios.

5. Tonfa:

• **Description:** The tonfa is a wooden weapon resembling a club with a handle. It is used primarily for striking and blocking techniques.

Techniques:

• **Strikes:** Practitioners can deliver powerful strikes using both ends of the tonfa, targeting various parts of the body.

• **Blocks:** The tonfa can effectively block incoming strikes, providing a defensive advantage.

- **Joint Locks:** The design allows for manipulation of the opponent's joints, enabling control techniques.

- **Applications:** Tonfa training develops coordination, timing, and understanding of angles. It is often practiced in forms and self-defense techniques.

Basic weapons training in Shaolin Kempo Karate provides practitioners with essential skills and techniques that enhance their martial arts proficiency. Each weapon offers unique benefits, contributing to the overall development of coordination, timing, and self-defense abilities.

By mastering these basic weapons, practitioners gain a deeper understanding of martial arts and its rich history, philosophy, and practical applications. Regular practice and study of these weapons will lead to improved skills, confidence, and appreciation for the art of Shaolin Kempo Karate.

Advanced Weapons Techniques

Advanced weapons techniques in Shaolin Kempo Karate build upon the foundational skills learned with basic weapons. Mastering these techniques requires a deep understanding of timing, precision, and fluidity of movement. Here's an overview of some advanced weapons techniques, including their descriptions, execution, and applications:

1. Bo Staff Techniques

A. Spinning Techniques:

• **Description:** Spinning the bo staff around the body can create distance, confuse opponents, and enhance control.

Execution:

• Begin with the staff held in one hand.

Use wrist movement to spin the staff, passing it from one hand to the other.

• Incorporate footwork to create angles and evade attacks.

Applications: Effective for both offense and defense, spinning techniques can create openings for strikes while providing a dynamic defensive maneuver.

B. Figure-Eight Patterns:

• **Description:** A figure-eight motion enhances fluidity and rhythm, allowing for both defensive and offensive applications.

Execution:

• Hold the staff at one end and move it in a figure-eight pattern around your body.

• Practice transitioning from offensive strikes to defensive blocks seamlessly.

Applications: This technique helps maintain distance while effectively striking or blocking against multiple opponents.

2. Nunchaku Techniques

A. Multiple Strikes:

• **Description:** Executing rapid combinations of strikes using the nunchaku can overwhelm an opponent.

Execution:

• Start with a basic strike and follow up with quick successive strikes to various target areas (head, ribs, legs).

• Incorporate spinning motions to maintain flow and create openings.

Applications: This technique is effective in sparring and self-defense, keeping opponents on the defensive and unable to counterattack.

B. Disarm Techniques:

• **Description:** Using the nunchaku to disarm an opponent's weapon.

Execution:

• Move in close to the opponent while maintaining control of your nunchaku.

• Use the chain to hook and pull the opponent's weapon away while simultaneously striking.

Applications: Disarming techniques can turn an opponent's attack against them, providing an opportunity for counterattacks.

3. Sai Techniques

A. Flipping Techniques:

• **Description:** Flipping the sai for rapid transitions between offensive and defensive moves.

Execution:

• Rotate the sai in hand while executing a thrust or strike.

• Use the flipping motion to transition quickly into blocking or trapping positions.

• **Applications:** This technique enhances agility and allows for quick responses to changing situations.

B. Combination Techniques

• **Description:** Using both sai simultaneously for fluid attacks and defenses.

Execution:

• Practice alternating strikes with each sai, creating a rhythm and flow.

• Incorporate traps and blocks with one sai while attacking with the other.

Applications: Combination techniques can keep opponents off-balance and create openings for follow-up attacks.

4. Katana Techniques

A. Iaijutsu (Quick Draw Techniques):

- **Description:** The art of drawing and cutting with the katana in a single motion.

Execution:

- Begin with the katana sheathed at your side.

- Practice drawing the blade while simultaneously executing a downward cut.

Applications: Iaijutsu techniques are effective for quick responses to surprise attacks, emphasizing speed and precision.

B. Mizukage (Water Shadow Technique):

- **Description:** A technique involving fluid movement and deceptive strikes.

Execution:

• Move in and out of range, feinting strikes to mislead your opponent.

• Use angles to create opportunities for unexpected cuts and thrusts.

Applications: This technique emphasizes adaptability and can be useful in both sparring and self-defense situations.

5. Tonfa Techniques:

A. Joint Locks and Manipulations

• **Description:** Using the tonfa to control an opponent through joint manipulation.

Execution:

• Position the tonfa against the opponent's joint (e.g., wrist or elbow).

- Apply pressure to create leverage, controlling their movement.

Applications: This technique can effectively immobilize an opponent, allowing for control and restraint.

B. Combination Strikes:

- **Description:** Using the tonfa to deliver rapid combinations of strikes.

Execution:

- Incorporate various angles and strikes, using both ends of the tonfa.

- Practice transitioning from strikes to blocks seamlessly.

Applications: Combination strikes can overwhelm opponents, providing opportunities for finishing techniques.

Advanced weapons techniques in Shaolin Kempo Karate enhance a practitioner's skills and understanding of martial arts. Mastery of these techniques requires dedication, precision, and regular practice.

By incorporating advanced techniques with fundamental skills, practitioners develop greater proficiency and confidence in using weapons effectively in self-defense, sparring, and forms. Regular training and application of these advanced techniques will lead to improved martial arts capabilities and a deeper appreciation for the art of Shaolin Kempo Karate.

CHAPTER 8: CONDITIONING AND STRENGTH TRAINING
Strength Training Exercises

Strength training is an essential component of martial arts training, including Shaolin Kempo Karate. It enhances overall physical fitness, improves technique execution, and increases power in strikes.

Below is a list of effective strength training exercises tailored for martial artists, focusing on functional strength, stability, and agility.

1. Bodyweight Exercises

A. Push-Ups:

• **Target Muscles:** Chest, shoulders, triceps, core

Execution:

• Start in a plank position with hands shoulder-width apart.

• Lower your body until your chest nearly touches the ground.

• Push back up to the starting position.

Variations: Incline push-ups, decline push-ups, and one-arm push-ups.

B. Squats:

• **Target Muscles:** Quadriceps, hamstrings, glutes, lower back

Execution:

• Stand with feet shoulder-width apart.

• Lower your body as if sitting back into a chair, keeping your chest up.

• Return to the starting position.

Variations: Jump squats, pistol squats, and sumo squats.

C. Lunges:

• **Target Muscles:** Quadriceps, hamstrings, glutes, calves

Execution:

• Stand with feet together, then step forward with one leg.

• Lower your hips until both knees are bent at about a 90-degree angle.

• Push back to the starting position and switch legs.

Variations: Reverse lunges, lateral lunges, and walking lunges.

2. Resistance Training:

A. Dumbbell Shoulder Press:

• **Target Muscles:** Shoulders, triceps, upper chest

Execution:

• Stand or sit with a dumbbell in each hand at shoulder height.

• Press the weights overhead until your arms are fully extended.

• Lower the weights back to shoulder height.

Variations: Arnold press and single-arm shoulder press.

B. Dumbbell Rows:

• **Target Muscles:** Back, biceps, shoulders

Execution:

• Bend at the hips with a dumbbell in each hand, keeping your back straight.

• Pull the dumbbells towards your waist, squeezing your shoulder blades together.

• Lower the weights back down.

Variations: Bent-over rows, single-arm rows, and renegade rows.

C. Deadlifts:

• **Target Muscles:** Hamstrings, glutes, lower back

Execution:

• Stand with feet hip-width apart, holding a barbell or dumbbells in front of you.

• Hinge at the hips and lower the weights towards the ground while keeping your back straight.

• Stand back up by engaging your glutes and hamstrings.

Variations: Romanian deadlifts, sumo deadlifts, and single-leg deadlifts.

3. Core Strength Exercises

A. Plank:

• **Target Muscles:** Core, shoulders, back

Execution:

• Start in a push-up position with elbows under your shoulders.

• Keep your body in a straight line from head to heels.

• Hold the position for a specified time.

Variations: Side plank, forearm plank, and plank with leg lifts.

B. Russian Twists:

• **Target Muscles:** Obliques, core

Execution:

• Sit on the ground with your knees bent and lean back slightly.

• Hold a weight or medicine ball and twist your torso to one side, then the other.

Variations: Feet on the ground, feet elevated, or using a heavier weight.

C. Leg Raises:

• **Target Muscles:** Lower abs, hip flexors

Execution:

• Lie on your back with legs straight.

• Lift your legs toward the ceiling while keeping them straight.

• Lower your legs back down without touching the ground.

Variations: Hanging leg raises, bent-knee raises, and flutter kicks.

4. Functional Strength Training

A. Kettlebell Swings:

• **Target Muscles:** Glutes, hamstrings, core, shoulders

Execution:

• Stand with feet shoulder-width apart, holding a kettlebell with both hands.

• Hinge at the hips to swing the kettlebell between your legs.

• Explode through your hips to swing the kettlebell up to shoulder height.

Variations: Single-arm kettlebell swings and double kettlebell swings.

B. Medicine Ball Throws:

• **Target Muscles:** Core, shoulders, chest

Execution:

• Stand with feet shoulder-width apart, holding a medicine ball at chest level.

• Twist your torso and throw the ball against a wall or to a partner.

Variations: Overhead throws and chest passes.

C. Battle Ropes:

• **Target Muscles:** Full body, focusing on shoulders, core, and legs

Execution:

• Stand with feet shoulder-width apart, holding a battle rope in each hand.

• Create waves in the ropes by rapidly moving your arms up and down or side to side.

Applications: Battle ropes enhance endurance, strength, and coordination.

Incorporating strength training exercises into your Shaolin Kempo Karate regimen enhances physical capabilities essential for martial arts. These exercises develop power, stability, and endurance, improving overall performance in techniques, forms, and sparring. Regularly incorporating these exercises, alongside your martial arts training, will lead to better strength, balance, and agility, contributing to your growth as a martial artist. Always ensure to practice proper form and technique to prevent injuries.

Developing Mental Focus And Discipline

Developing mental focus and discipline is essential for success in martial arts, including Shaolin Kempo Karate. Mental strength enhances performance, aids in mastering techniques, and improves overall well-being. Here are several strategies and practices to cultivate mental focus and discipline in your martial arts journey:

1. Mindfulness Meditation

A. Practice Regularly:

• Set aside time each day for mindfulness meditation, even if it's just for 5-10 minutes.

• Find a quiet space, sit comfortably, and focus on your breath. Allow thoughts to come and go without judgment.

B. Benefits:

• Enhances concentration and awareness, helping you stay present during training.

• Reduces stress and anxiety, promoting a calm mindset.

2. Goal Setting

A. Define Clear Goals:

• Set specific, measurable, achievable, relevant, and time-bound (SMART) goals for your martial arts training.

• Break down larger goals into smaller, manageable steps to track progress.

B. Benefits:

• Provides a clear focus for your training sessions.

• Helps maintain motivation and commitment to your practice.

3. Visualization Techniques

A. Mental Imagery:

• Spend time visualizing yourself successfully executing techniques, forms, or sparring scenarios.

• Picture every detail, including your movements, environment, and feelings of accomplishment.

B. Benefits:

• Strengthens neural pathways related to the skills you're practicing, improving actual performance.

• Builds confidence and reduces anxiety before competitions or sparring.

4. Breath Control

A. Breathing Exercises:

• Practice deep breathing exercises to calm the mind and body.

• Inhale deeply through the nose, hold for a moment, and exhale slowly through the mouth.

B. Benefits:

• Helps manage stress and anxiety, enhancing focus during training.

• Promotes relaxation and clarity, improving overall performance.

5. Consistent Training Routine

A. Establish a Schedule: Create a training schedule that includes both physical practice and mental exercises.

• Stick to the schedule, treating each session as an essential commitment.

B. Benefits

• Fosters discipline through consistent practice.

• Builds muscle memory and mental resilience over time.

6. Positive Affirmations

A. Use Affirmations:

• Develop positive affirmations that reinforce your goals and abilities (e.g., "I am focused and disciplined in my training").

• Repeat these affirmations daily to boost confidence and maintain a positive mindset.

B. Benefits:

• Helps combat negative self-talk and builds a resilient mindset.

• Encourages a growth-oriented approach to challenges in your training.

7. Focus on Technique

A. Mindful Practice:

• During training, focus solely on the technique you are practicing.

• Eliminate distractions and dedicate your attention to executing movements correctly.

B. Benefits:

• Improves skill mastery and retention.

• Enhances overall performance by developing a deeper understanding of techniques.

8. Journaling

A. Reflective Journaling:

• Keep a training journal to record your thoughts, progress, challenges, and insights.

• Reflect on your training sessions and set intentions for future practice.

B. Benefits:

• Provides clarity on your mental and physical progress.

• Helps identify areas for improvement and maintain focus on goals.

9. Engage in Challenges:

A. Push Your Limits:

• Regularly challenge yourself with new techniques, sparring partners, or training environments.

• Embrace discomfort as a way to grow and develop resilience.

B. Benefits:

• Builds mental toughness and adaptability.

• Enhances problem-solving skills and focus under pressure.

10. Seek Guidance

A. Mentorship and Support:

• Work with a coach, instructor, or experienced practitioner who can provide guidance and support.

• Engage in group classes or training sessions to foster camaraderie and accountability.

B. Benefits:

• Offers a structured approach to developing focus and discipline.

• Encourages a supportive community that reinforces your commitment to growth.

Developing mental focus and discipline in Shaolin Kempo Karate is a multifaceted process that involves regular practice, self-reflection, and the implementation of various techniques.

By incorporating mindfulness, goal setting, visualization, and other strategies into your training regimen, you will enhance your mental strength, improve performance, and cultivate a deeper connection to your martial arts practice. Consistency and perseverance are key; the more you invest in your mental development, the greater your progress will be on the mat and in life.

Conclusion

The journey of mastering Shaolin Kempo Karate extends beyond physical techniques; it encompasses mental focus, discipline, and holistic development. By integrating strength training, advanced techniques, and mental conditioning practices such as mindfulness, goal setting, and visualization, practitioners can cultivate a well-rounded martial arts experience.

Developing mental focus and discipline not only enhances performance in training and competitions but also promotes resilience and a positive mindset in everyday life. Consistent practice, self-reflection, and engagement with supportive mentors and communities further reinforce this growth.

Ultimately, the principles and practices of Shaolin Kempo Karate offer valuable lessons in perseverance, self-awareness, and personal growth. Embracing this journey will lead to improved skills, increased confidence, and a deeper appreciation for the art of martial arts, enriching both your practice and your life. Stay dedicated to your training, and let the lessons learned through Shaolin Kempo Karate guide you on your path to excellence.

Glossary Of Terms

Here's a glossary of common terms used in Shaolin Kempo Karate, which can help practitioners and enthusiasts better understand the art and its concepts:

- **Adrenaline Dump:** The release of adrenaline in response to a stressful situation, often affecting physical performance and mental clarity during combat.
- **Bo:** A long wooden staff, typically 6 feet in length, used in traditional martial arts.
- **Chamber:** The position in which a weapon or limb is held before executing a strike or technique.
- **Disarm:** The act of taking a weapon away from an opponent.
- **Elbow Strike:** A close-range striking technique using the elbow.

- **Focus Mitts:** Pads worn by a trainer to facilitate striking practice for students.

- **Grappling:** Close-quarters fighting techniques focused on holds, throws, and joint locks.

- **Hana:** A Japanese term for "flower," often used metaphorically to describe beauty in movement.

- **Iaijutsu:** The art of drawing the sword and cutting in one motion.

- **Joint Lock:** A technique used to control an opponent by applying pressure to a joint, restricting movement.

- **Kata:** A pre-arranged sequence of movements and techniques used for practice and demonstration.

- **Lunge:** A stepping technique used to close distance or evade an attack.

- **Meditation:** A mental practice aimed at achieving a state of focused relaxation and heightened awareness.

- **Nunchaku:** A traditional weapon consisting of two sticks connected by a chain or rope, often used for striking and trapping.

- **Oss:** A term of respect used among martial artists, often expressing acknowledgment or greeting.

- **Pressure Points:** Specific points on the body that, when struck or manipulated, can cause pain or incapacitation.

- **Qi (Chi):** A concept in traditional Chinese culture referring to vital energy or life force.

- **Rei:** A Japanese term for bowing, demonstrating respect to instructors and fellow practitioners.

- **Sparring:** Controlled practice fighting between practitioners to develop skills and techniques in a realistic setting.

- **Throw:** A technique used to unbalance an opponent and bring them to the ground.

- **Uke:** The receiving practitioner in a technique or sparring scenario.

- **Visualization:** A mental practice where practitioners envision themselves successfully executing techniques or achieving goals.

- **Weapons Training:** The practice of using various traditional weapons to enhance martial skills.

- **X-factor:** A unique quality or skill that sets a practitioner apart, often referring to their individual style or approach.

- **Yoko:** A Japanese term meaning "side," often used in reference to lateral movements or techniques.

- **Zen:** A school of Mahayana Buddhism that emphasizes meditation and mindfulness, often influencing martial arts philosophy.

It is crucial for practitioners of Shaolin Kempo Karate to have a solid understanding of these phrases since it has the potential to improve communication, comprehension of methods, and the entire experience of practicing martial arts. The purpose of this glossary is to provide students of all levels with a helpful resource that will assist them on their quest toward ultimate mastery of the art.

ABOUT THE AUTHOR:

Kameron Jalen, an author, frequently employs his profound comprehension of human nature and personal experiences to investigate a diverse array of themes in his writing. His compositions may encompass instructional materials, non-fiction, or fiction, which demonstrate his capacity to articulate intricate concepts in a manner that is both engaging and comprehensible. Jalen's objective in his writing is to motivate and inspire readers by imparting knowledge on the significance of personal development, self-discipline, and resilience.

Kameron Jalen is also a dedicated martial arts practitioner, having trained in a variety of disciplines. His proficiency in martial arts is not only indicative of his physical abilities, but also underscores the philosophical and cerebral components of the discipline. He is likely to promote the advantages of martial arts in the development of focus, discipline, and confidence, and he may conduct seminars or teach classes to disseminate his expertise. He integrates the principles of hard work and perseverance into both his writing and teaching, as evidenced by his martial arts journey.

Kameron Jalen has a Ph.D. in a pertinent discipline from a prestigious university in the United States, in addition to his creative and physical activities. His academic education equips him with a robust foundation for his writing and teaching, enabling him to approach subjects with a critical and analytical perspective. His scholarly work and research may concentrate on the social implications of martial arts, human behavior, or psychology, thereby contributing to both academic discourse and practical applications.

Kameron Jalen possesses an uncommon combination of academic rigor, physical prowess, and creativity. He remains a source of inspiration and influence for those in his vicinity, motivating them to pursue their interests and aspire for excellence in all aspects of life because of his diverse talents. Jalen is dedicated to the promotion of personal and professional development, whether through his academic lectures, martial arts classes, or publications.

THE END